CONTENTS

1. MY STORY 8

2. WHY ARE WE SO FAT, UNHEAL
AND UNHAPPY? 22

3. ABS ARE MADE IN THE KITCHEN,
DISEASE STARTS IN YOUR GUT. 29

4. MEN ARE STUPID. 37

5. EAT FAT. 47

6. SO WHAT DO I EAT TO PISS THIS GLITTER 52

7. WHAT ABOUT A MEAL PLAN? 93

8. THREE WEEK GUT CHECK 103

9. THREE STEPS TO STEMS AND ABS 114

10. THREE WEEKS OF SWEAT 124

11. RECIPES 155

12. RESOURCES 179

13. REFERENCES 182

COPYRIGHT

DISCLAIMER

Eat clean. Piss glitter. Workout guide, recipes, and all components included are not medical advice and are not intended to replace the advice or attention of healthcare professionals. Always consult your physician before beginning or making any changes into your diet and/or exercise program, for diagnosis and treatment of illness and injuries, and for advice regarding medications.

Disclaimer: You must get your physician's approval before making any changes to your diet and/or exercise program including every step discussed in this guide. These recommendations are not medical guidelines, but for educational purposes only. You must consult your physician prior to taking any advice from this program/manual or if you have any medical condition or injury that contraindicates physical activity or supplementation. This advice is intended for healthy individuals 18 years and older only.

The information in this program is meant to supplement, not replace, proper exercise training and nutrition along with the approval of your physician. All forms of exercise and nutrition pose inherent risks. The author advises all readers to take full responsibility for their safety, know their limits, and seek expert guidance for performing all exercises contained within this guide. Exercises and dietary recommendations are not intended as a substitute for any exercise routine or treatment or dietary regimen that may have been prescribed by your physician.

See your physician before starting any exercise or nutrition program or making any changes. If you are taking any medication, you must talk to your physician before starting any exercise program, including any recommendations in this program. If you experience lightheadedness, dizziness, or shortness of breath while exercising, stop the movement and consult a physician immediately. Do not perform any exercise unless you have been shown the proper technique by a certified personal trainer or certified strength and conditioning specialist. Always ask for instruction and assistance when lifting. Do not perform any exercise without proper instruction. Always warm up prior to strength training and interval training.

You must have a complete physical examination if you are sedentary, have high cholesterol, high blood pressure, or diabetes, if you are overweight, if you have had any injuries, may have an injury, or if you are over 30 years old. Please discuss all nutritional changes with your physician or a registered dietician. If your physician recommends that you do not use any information in this program, please follow your doctor's orders. This information is intended for informational use only. Whitney Benjamin and hiitters inc. LLC will not assume any liability or be held responsible for any form of injury, personal loss, or illness caused by the utilization of this information.

In addition, make sure you use equipment that is properly maintained and safe. You must also have the exercises taught to you by a certified personal trainer or strength coach and have a spotter with you during exercises. Please note, affiliate links are used for recommended products.

Although every precaution has been taken to verify the accuracy of the information contained herein, the author and publisher assume no responsibility for any errors or omissions. No liability is assumed for damages that may result from the use of information contained within.

CONTACT AND MORE INFORMATION

Whitney Benjamin beezybodyfit@gmail.com

Photography by: Michelle Mattox Photography and Design

Cover Design and Styling by: Kylie Lazo

Hair by: Julie Withers

Interior Design by: Whitney Benjamin

Editor: Robin Canedy

Book Consultant: Savannah Brown

Publisher: Whitney Benjamin

ISBN - 978-1503193703

Health, Fitness, Nutrition, Paleo, Workout plans, Women's Health, Women's Fitness

DEDICATION

This is for Wubbas, may you always be full of joy and wonder.

This is for Bubs, may you always guide, nurture and be my home.

This is for my mom, may you always be my rock, my roots and guide my wings.

This is for my dad, may you always be our strength and build our dreams.

This is for my brother, may you always be humble, kind and teach your nature to my son.

Without these souls, this guide does not exist.

I tend to get lost, but you all are my compass.

My cup runneth over.

ACKNOWLEDGEMENTS

Thank you to my husband for letting me to "create" as a career. And more, for believing that I could.

Thank you to Savannah Rose for believing, editing and cheering me on every step of the way.

Thank you to Robin Canedy for keeping me streamlined, focused and edited.

Thank you to my ridiculously amazing and selfless mom for watching Wubbas anytime I just needed a few hours to write, sweat or be alone.

Thank you to Michelle Mattox for bringing this book to life with her beautiful images, talent and inspiration.

Thank you to January Newland for being my witch mother, and helping me learn to love and nourish my body from the inside out.

Thank you to Kylie Lazo for her amazing styling support and design of the cover.

Thank you to Julie Withers for my big, gorgeous and fabulous hair.

Thank you to the Coffee & Tea Collective for giving me an office with a view and delightful espresso to fuel my words.

BE MERRY COMMANDMENTS

Be fiercely protective of your time and graciously conscious of others'.

Time is all we have. It feels like forever but looking back it never really is. Your loved ones may or may not be here tomorrow. You may not be here tomorrow.

Learn to say no to things that do not make you happy or bring prosperity to your family. Our time is valuable and we must protect it. If you give it away you will never learn your value, so how could anyone else?

Become a researcher of your own well-being.

Something that works for one will not work for all. I will say it again and again and again— everyBODY is different, so you have to keep trying new things until the mix is right for you.

Guilt and joy cannot coexist.

Enjoy life. There are going to be times you have to cheat on yourself and your diet, if you want to call it that. Enjoy every bite.

Guilt is where we continue to punish ourselves and make the same mistakes over and over again because we are already in the pity party boat, and it's easier to keep rowing than to jump out and swim to shore.

Swim to shore, and enjoy the taste of salt water while you are at it

Inspire change in others with the change in yourself.

This lesson sucks. I want to tell everyone I love why the food and habits around them are unhealthy, but it will always fall upon deaf ears unless they seek me out and are actually ready to change.

As humans, we respond much better to change we can see than change we simply hear about. Do not force change on others, but inspire change with how much you are rocking at life.

Harm no one. Be nice to yourself.

In the practice of Wicca, one of the most current and known forms of witchcraft, karma is a big factor in what the universe deals you— karma onto others and karma onto yourself. "Harm ye none and do what ye will," is their belief. It basically means so long as your actions bring no harm on others AND YOURSELF, live freely, act freely, and move freely.

I learned this in high school but never practiced it until I found myself pregnant. I was always kind to others but not myself.

Pregnancy changed me. It allowed me to find love within myself; perhaps, I just grew into a mother that knew nourishment started within. In any case, learn and practice it now. Love and be kind to others, but always start with yourself.

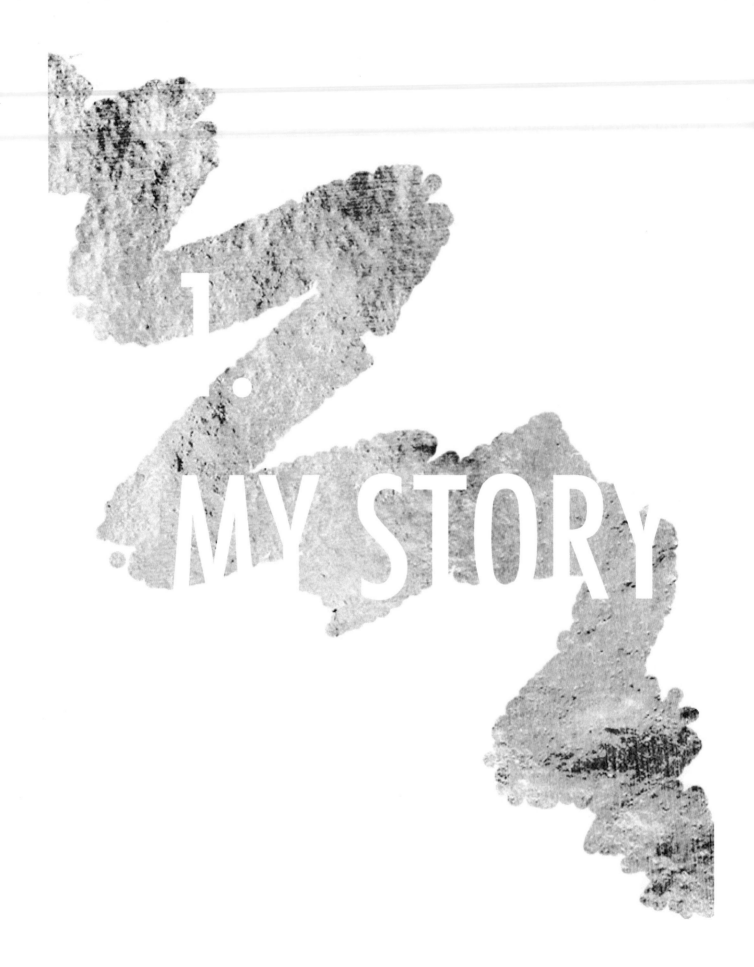

1.
MY STORY

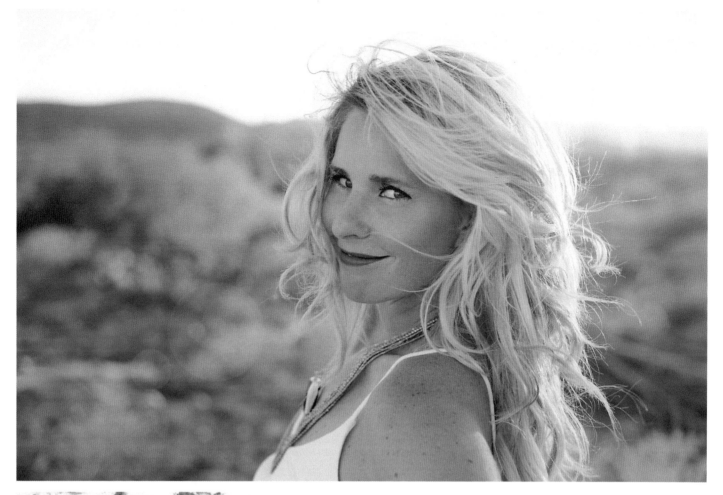

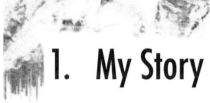

1. My Story

Why I rant

To be honest, I doubted myself in writing this book, this guide, this how-to, this whatever you want to call it. Who am I to write a book about healthy living?

This question plagued my efforts and still causes me the occasional hiccup. My bu-thigh (where the donk meets the back of your thigh) has cellulite. My thighs rubs. My arms jiggle. My abs however, are great.

I have never been accused of being too thin; in fact, I am allergic to it.

I thought I was too normal to write this. My breakthrough moment was in talking about my fears with a few good girlfriends—my coven, if you will.

Thank God for them. They are to me what cappuccinos are to my writing—soul nourishment, brain fuel.

One friend said to me, "Who is anyone to write a book about nutrition and working out? There are only so many 'new' ideas out there. It is all about the delivery. Your story is worth sharing, and if it helps even one person, it's worth it."

In this moment, I crashed my own pity party and started pouring my life into something real.

Being too normal is exactly why I needed to put pen to paper. I am not cashing in on good genetics or luck. I work my ass off to look somewhat acceptable in a two-piece. Health has broken my heart one too many times, and if I can spare some heartbreak, I am all in.

This. Just. In. What I will tell you about nutrition and fitness is not new. I did not invent this way of life; I simply hacked my own life until I found what worked. This is a process I think anyone who seeks permanent change really has to go through.

What I hope to save you in your process is much of the self-inflicted emotional and physical pain that I endured. The pain I still endure, really, because my battle is on going.

I am not a nutritionist or registered dietician, for one, and I am not convinced a program exists that could certify my beliefs when it comes to nutrition. Most nutrition degrees are rooted in the USDA's food pyramid, and it is not much more than a pyramid scheme to keep big business in business and the rest of us fat.

However, it is quite possible that I am certifiably insane when it comes to what I put in my body. The last decade of my life has, in large part, been dedicated to reading, researching, and experimenting on my own body through nutrition and fitness. I have read thousands—I mean THOUSANDS—of articles, books and studies, mapping out my own mind-numbing syllabus in health and wellness.

If I had a dollar for every time along the way my boyfriend turned husband has told me I am crazy for refusing to eat something or demanding to, well I'd be sitting on a yacht in Ibiza writing this book.

But, in my madness I found sanity. Through nutrition I have beaten disease, fought infertility, and, most importantly, found a love for my body that never existed, and sadly for most women never will. It is the madness and the love I aim to share with you.

Kindness Within

I hope you walk away from reading my rant questioning everything you can about your own health. Trust no one (entirely-blindly), but listen to their reasoning.

Don't even trust me. Everybody is different, unique, and complex to which no one diet or workout will fit a universal prescription.

Be a student of your own health, love your body, and remember you only get one.

I can hear you chewing that over. Love your body . . . you've heard it over and over again. You've seen it on Instagram. You've heard beautiful "skinny" beezies scream it from the rooftops.

Quite frankly, you're sick of it. I get it. You're thinking, sure, I will love my body as soon as I have a body I like.

The reality is that you have to start treating your body with love and kindness to ever achieve the body you like, let alone love.

In love and kindness, we nourish and take care of others. We see to their needs. We want them to be optimally healthy and thriving. It is the same within our own souls. We simply get lost in how to apply our own medicine.

If you cannot love your body today in this moment, at least stop talking shit about it. Stop reminding it of that (insert wrinkle, chub rub, piece of cellulite, skin flap, brown spot, crooked tooth) that no one notices but you.

Kindness within is your first and most important goal.

Kindness within is the new goal weight.

Your Body, Your Responsibility

It is seeing my insecure 7th grade self in most of the young female athletes I work with on a daily basis that served as the impetus for writing this. My mission is to teach women, and anyone who will listen really, that you are 100% in charge of your health and that it starts with what you decide to put in your body.

Sometimes we are unlucky in health and in life. Sometimes we have a chance to avoid the icky things. Sometimes we do not.
I learned a very tough lesson when I was fourteen. People die—people you love, people who are too young, people who had much to serve to the world, people who make you a better person today.

I lost my first little love, Johnny Villani. He was full of laughter and hope, despite his world of daily injections, oxygen tanks, and hoping for an organ transplant to save his life from cystic fibrosis.

He lost his battle a couple of weeks after my fourteenth birthday, a birthday on which he sent me a dozen yellow roses from his hospital room and vowed to send me a dozen red roses the next year when we would, of course, be in love.

To this day, I wonder who he would be, who we would be. He had enough laughter for the world, was a gifted golfer, and a smart ass. Just like me. We were perfect.

I miss him. This book is for him. He taught me that you cannot take your health for granted. He taught me that you cannot take those you love for granted. While Johnny was dealt an unlucky hand of genetics, I will forever be militant regarding my health and that of my family, because it is our responsibility to prevent what we can.

My mission is woven with parts of Johnny: Seek health. Seek laughter. Seek now.

Society will not teach you how to eat. Society will trick you into devouring years of Fiber One bars, storing fat, and developing chronic diseases as a result of poor digestion and inflammation.

It is officially your responsibility to prevent poor health from developing in your body because sometimes disease can be avoided. Sometimes disease can subside.

Always, we have a choice to give our bodies the best chance to thrive. Do what you can.

My Insane Path to Sanity

The road I walked to wellness, and quite frankly the best abs I've ever known, was paved with major falls and big leaps. Not like scraping both knees kind of falling. I am talking about knocking out my front teeth kind of falling. Falls that took me to dark places.

Places where I was afraid to look in the mirror. Places where I would have judged myself terribly. Luckily, I have always been surrounded with tremendous love and support from my family, both blood and love related, and was always able to find my way home.

Without their love, I would still be on the road hitchhiking my way through before and after photos, in pain, chubs a rubbing, and alone.

As much as I would like this to be my journey and to be able to do everything on my own, my shortcomings always remind me that it is a journey shared with those I love.

Enough mush; shall we get real? In 6th grade when I had to change for PE in front of other little beezies, my best friend Brittany taught me how to suck in my belly to look skinnier.

USELESS NOTE:

We somehow acquired the nickname "Shittney twins" along the way.

Then sometime in 7th grade, they weighed us to see where we landed in the old sliding fat percentiles. I remember telling my friends, "I weigh 115." And my frienemy Jessica said, "Ohhh, my God!" She then proceeded to grab my belly and say, "Hopefully, one day this will go to your boobs!"

This was the terrible wretched aha moment that triggered hatred for my body. I stepped on that scale thinking nothing of my weight and stepped off questioning every bite.

To this day, I hate when people touch my stomach, even my hubs, though I believe my self-awareness is letting this go little by little. The point is, in 7th grade it had begun. I was twelve, and I was fat because I had a tummy and had not yet grown into my body.

I was in no way actually fat, but in my head and to Jessica, I was fat and that is all that mattered. It is really easy to walk your belief into reality. It happens in seconds and takes years to erase. This one little moment of one little beezy being a beezy is where my journey of ~~wanting~~ obsessing over a better body began. And so it begins for too many girls.

In high school, I learned if you ate basically nothing you would be skinny. Great, because I have always, ALWAYS had a donk, and being slender has never easy for me.

When my high school boyfriend and the "dream school" recruiting me for softball both ate my heart, shat it out, lit it on fire, and stomped on it, I found myself to be borderline anorexic. But, I was skinny, so that was a win in my book! It was a skinny lesson that proved to be fat in emotional and physical damage by the end.

12

Fast forward to my first quarter at my true dream school UCLA, and let's discuss the freshmen ~~fifteen~~ twenty-five pounds that assaulted me due to a huge amount of weightlifting, and having no clue how to fuel my body.

A typical day looked like this:

- Wake up for conditioning or weights at the literal butt crack of dawn.
- Breakfast of a Pop-Tart, or a huge HEALTHY bowl of oatmeal brown sugar, fruit, or a waffle (or four waffles depending on if it was a conditioning day).
- Class or nap (most likely a nap since I went to class bi-quarterly for the midterm and final).
- Skipped lunch or had a sandwich if I was starving, opted for a diet Rockstar
- Hours of practice heading into afternoon/evening/sometimes night time depending on our team's effort and our coaches' moods that day.
- Chowing down multiple, multiple bowls of Rice Krispies or Kashi cereal (for the whole grains) at dinner, and probably a side of French fries, oh and a side salad to be healthy.
- Shower. Sleep immediately. Repeat the next day.
- Midterm or final weeks sometimes meant bathing in copious amounts of diet Rockstar, caffeine pills, eating nothing, studying all night, and basically starving myself.

My body was storing fat, aching with so much pain, and I could not for the life of me figure out why.

I was working my donk off! Now I know my body was starving for nutrients, craving rest, and was truly chronically dehydrated. It is no wonder that by the end of my freshmen year I had developed full blown rheumatoid arthritis (RA). Which is basically an autoimmune condition where your body attacks its own joints because it believes there is an infection there.

I was barely able to grip the bat, and the condition severely hindered my agility, speed, and overall zest for life. Taking upwards of eight pills a day simply to function, I had gained fifteen pounds in excess fat and bloat due the mix of icky chemicals and toxic ingredients in my medicine.

The disease stole all of my energy. I was depressed and ready to walk away from the game I loved, as I could no longer work out with my team at the capacity everyone else could, and the pain was crippling.

The months following my RA diagnosis were a dark and low time for me. I was chunky. There were days I just couldn't get out of bed and head down to the weight room. I had to get up an hour earlier and soak in the bathtub just to loosen up my joints and put weight on my feet without wincing in pain every step.

I wanted to quit softball—the only true life love I had known—and I could not be bothered to walk two blocks to dinner. I would rather drive in LA traffic and fight parking than walk.

It was in the summer that followed when I hit rock bottom and blossomed the most. I smoked a lot of weed.

I realize now I was self-medicating for the physical and emotional pain the diagnosis created, but it is not a pretty time in my life I like to recall.

It is difficult even typing the words and admitting it now. Very few friends have ever seen that side of my life, the side I hide that makes me seem anything less than perfect. I wish you could sit in my skin with me as I cringe imagining my parents, coach, and loved ones feeling defeated a bit in that admittance.

::I feel it is important to add that before this summer, I was pretty straight edge. I had maybe smoked a couple of times and was always terrified of doing the wrong thing, or sacrificing my career and reputation for that matter. That is why admitting it now, literally, is a punch in the gut. However, I am a firm believer that a punch in the gut is just a pause so you can catch your breath and grow. So I am doing my best to revel in this pain right now as I type.::

The truth is, and he doesn't even know it, my husband saved me from myself. I met him in the middle of the summer, away from my binge of smoking bowls and on the edge of throwing away my softball career.

We were not dating, and I am not even sure he was really interested. I met him at a family BBQ, and I wanted to be a woman he would marry—the girl who enrolled at UCLA with big dreams.

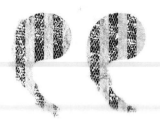

I am a firm believer that a punch in the gut is just a pause so you can catch your breath and grow.

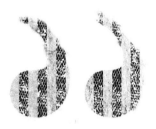

So, I stopped smoking and started running. I wanted to be in shape for softball, but I really wanted to be in shape for him, or even the idea of him because he still really did not know I existed.

Running miles and miles and miles, eating two protein shakes a day and a salad with a little bit of chicken for dinner, I was finally skinny. SUCCESS was mine for a couple of months at least!

School started in the fall; handsome and I fell in love; I got busy with team workouts and class, stopped running on my own, and gained some of the poundage right back—real quick.

"The fuck?" I said to myself in the mirror.

"Where did my abs go? All I had to eat today was a bowl of oatmeal, a South Beach Diet bar, a Diet Rockstar, and like three bowls of organic Panda Puffs. I squatted a good 170 pounds this morning, we ran a ton at practice, and I have a food baby!"

What was happening to me happens to a lot of female athletes. I followed a workout routine prescribed from the football team's strength coach, created a lot of muscle, and as a result was constantly feeling starved.

Quick science break:

Muscle is quite possibly the greediest of all your metabolic parts. Meaning (and I am really oversimplifying here) more muscle translates to more hunger due to more energy demands on your body.

Our team nutritionist told me I needed more whole grains and Gatorade, so I showered in that shit! Between morning weights and afternoon practices, I was on my feet for an average of at least six hours a day.

If I could calculate my calories, I would say I came in around 1,700 calories every day, which is not much for someone who is that active.

If the calorie is a calorie is a calorie rule is gospel, I should not have gained weight. I should have lost it. I lost weight in the summer by consuming less and burning more via cardio.

But what's important to note is that I did not just lose fat that summer; I lost muscle. My body was not recognizing my South Beach Diet bars and Diet Rockstars as nutrients, couldn't burn through all the organic carbs, and became a fat-storing machine as it tried to rebuild the muscle I lost.

What it boils down to is, I lost muscle tissue, water weight, and a little fat by eating less, running more, and by stopping my strength routine during the summer. As a result, my body's ability to store and burn glycogen was severely compromised.

Starving myself and excessive cardio was not a combination I could sustain. In stopping and adding back a weight routine, I ballooned up, which I believe most women would consider "bulking" up.

Too many carbs + Heavy lifting = bulk
Eating clean + Lots of protein + Lifting = haute

Fuck the System

Truth be told, the system failed me because there was never a holistic view of what was happening in my body. Everything was dissected into parts. Softball training meant heavy lifting.

Old school nutritionist meant showering in refined carbohydrates.

Specialist doctors meant treating a symptom with medicine (that hosted their own reactions), but never treating the entire human.

This was a combination that led to fat storage, inflammation, and depression.

Holistically, I was suffering as each part of my being was treated as isolated incidences.

Bulky and in pain, I began wondering how to get rid of arthritis. The chub was the least of my worries; I just wanted to feel good again.

Then my greatest aha moment came sitting in my rheumatologist's office staring at his huge, huge gut and cluttered desk and thinking to myself, What does this man know about health? How can he take care of me if he clearly has trouble taking care of himself?

He kept telling me, "Let's up your dosage. Your rheumatoid factor is the same or climbing," or "We just cannot be sure. Next step is injections!"

No. No. No. No. No. There is another way; there has to be. This bitch jumped out of the ear piercing chair about a dozen times before that happened; I am not about to inject something into myself every day to function.

It was in this moment I became a researcher and scientist of my own health. I donned a proverbial white coat and started researching every single thing I could in relation to RA, and the common denominator was food.

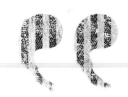

It was in this moment I became a researcher of my own health.

In my search for help, I read somewhere that sugars, chemicals, antibiotics, and toxins found in our meats and processed food led to inflammation and autoimmune disease. Then I read literally every book and article I could find on inflammation and nutrition and came to the conclusion that my diet consisting of daily Rice Krispies, processed everything, junky meat, white breads, and lots of sugar could be to blame for my RA.

I adapted a vegan whole-food based diet, and within one week every single symptom I had for RA was completely gone.

To my delight, so were my pills.

It is only looking back at the sequence of events that I can hypothesize what really happened within my body. In cutting out all processed foods and sugars, excessive carbohydrates, and crappy meat, I allowed my body to react to insulin appropriately. This slowly would have helped heal my gut and clear my body of inflammation that was causing the arthritis.

My gut was finally healthy again, but at the time, I had no idea how important the health of my gut really was. I have always heard that every disease, every illness starts in your gut, but now I know how very true this old wisdom is.

For a while, I ate mostly fresh greens and fruits, but was ALWAYS hungry and quickly became a "carb-a-terian."

Putting anything in my mouth on the accepted vegan list that would give me a jolt of energy, because in hindsight my nutrients were lacking, I was not getting enough proteins or fats and was replacing them with anything that would break down to sugar.

But boy, was I was loving me lots of soy based products and whole wheat everything.

Mmmm . . . soy, soy, soy, lots of mucus and extra estrogen! It kind of makes successive sense with my diet now consisting of fruit (sugar), whole wheat anything (sugar + difficult to break down), soy (mucus) and a few veggies (yay!), that three years ago I started to feel "off" again.

I lost my period for about a year and a half after stopping birth control, was diagnosed with polycystic ovary syndrome (PCOS) and was told my chances of having children without the help of drugs or treatment were pretty slim. I was handed a prescription for some hormones and sent on my merry way.

In short, PCOS is a pretty annoying disease. Full of abdominal cramping, irregular periods, outrageous acne, facial hair, and is known to be one of the leading causes of infertility. Killer!

Rock Bottom, Again.

If you ever want to cut a woman real, REAL deep, tell her she might not be able to have a child. This alone turned me into an alcoholic for a few months. My breaking point came on a WEDNESDAY morning ten minutes before I was supposed to be at work.

I sat in the shower dry heaving the bottle of champagne I drank alone the night before. Sitting down, sobbing, and faintly remembering the tough love talk my hubs gave me after I drove home drunk. Not a little drunk. Should have gone to jail drunk. We could call this rock bottom moment number two.

Sitting in that tub, I realized I had a choice. I could keep crying and self-medicating with champagne, or I could be the woman my hubs actually married and who my parents raised me to be, and deal with it head on.

Having walked the path of pills before, I refused to take more artificial hormones, already convinced the reason I had found my way to PCOS was due to my soy-based-sugar-laden diet and years of popping birth control pills. I healed myself through food once; it had to be possible again.

I dried out my champagne soaked white coat and once again began reading everything I could on ovarian cysts, reproductive health, and food, and again my diet changed. This time, the take home message was more nutrients, more healthy fats, and finding my way to superb gut health.

As a vegetarian, I was never getting enough nutrients because I was too concerned with getting full and never consuming fat soluble vitamins and minerals found in healthy meats.

Suddenly being "infertile," I felt in my bones that I needed meat again. I did not know I was missing nutrients and how much my body just cannot tolerate sugar. I just felt off and luckily stumbled upon the meaty change I needed.

Looking back and feeling how my body reacts now, I know that my body simply does not do well with a lot of sugar, and my vegetarian diet was drowning in it. Well, glucose broken down from all my carbs, not just traditional white sugar as you may be thinking of.

I will never forget the day my hubs made me the most delightful organic free-range chicken wings to break out of my vegetarian slump.

I told him I feel like I need to eat meat again. My body told me I needed it again.

So being the delightful chef he is, hubs made me the most perfect chicken wings to enjoy while watching a UCLA football game on our deck.

I will never forget the look on his face. He may have been more excited watching my first bite than he was proposing or marrying me. And though I was terrified of that bite, I immediately felt a sense of pressure release from my shoulders.

For years, I killed myself in what had become an elimination diet. What could I abstain from next? What detox would bring me closer to my goal weight?

It was a dangerous diet that terrorized my mind, agonized my body and soul. To this day, I wrestle that old dragon.

My handsome's love, along with the support of my coven, helps me find a path to wellness worth its weight in gold.

It truly is amazing what a little love does for someone. My hubs always puts so much love into his food, and I really needed his nourishment on this one.

My chicken wings were seasoned to perfection with just enough charred crisp on the edges for me to get lost in them. They were grilled, not fried like the batch he made for the rest of the party, and he once again saved me from myself.

After six years of being a vegetarian, I slowly adapted and now follow a whole-food based primal/paleo-ish diet. This way of noshing includes high quality organic meats, good quality fats like BUTTER, fruits and vegetables, no grains, daily pieces of dark chocolate, and, of course, gelato washed down with champagne on Sundays here and again.

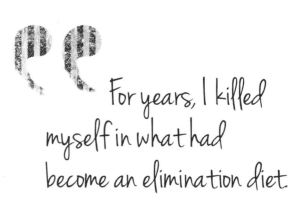

For years, I killed myself in what had become an elimination diet.

I like to say that I am a paleo-ish bitch who wears lipstick AND deodorant. I included daily tablespoons of apple cider vinegar into my regimen, experimented with coconut oil, and within two months of eating meat, I was barefoot, preggers, and gnawing on a piece of bacon.

The hubs who fought me HARD for not taking the hormones my doctor prescribed is now convinced that it was the introduction of meat that got me knocked up. I think it was a combination of good protein, healthy fats, controlling my blood sugar, nutrients . . . and coconut oil.

Perhaps, time just ran its course, but in following the diet I follow now, I have never in my life felt better. I gained little weight during my pregnancy, and my little Wubbas is as healthy as can be.

Long story long, I share my journey not to say that all medicine is bad and everything can be healed with food and natural witchcraft-ery. I share my story because the most valuable lesson I've learned is that you are in charge of your health, and simple changes in your diet can and will pay off immensely.

If something does not feel right, we pop a pill to make it better. I hate this behavior in my bones. I believe we have to find out why something doesn't feel right and treat the cause, not the symptom. Today, we see specialists for what we believe are isolated occurrences in our body, but they almost always are interconnected both in body and in mind. Even if it takes you days, months, or years to learn this lesson in practice, hear and believe it—now.

Newton's Law:

For every action, there is an equal and opposite reaction.

For every pill we consume, it creates a reaction in our body; some good and some that are very bad. For every bite we take, it creates a reaction of energy usage, energy storage, and all too often harm.

Food can cause your body to attack its own tissue, which is the case for all autoimmune conditions, and is the case for my body. Although everybody is very, very different, food really should be seen as medicine. Though I am no doctor, I will always write my own prescriptions in my kitchen and allow modern medicine to intervene when necessary.

Being healthy, looking good, and most importantly feeling good does not come easy to me. I struggle with it every single day. I was not blessed with genetics that give me effortless, long, and lean muscles.

Some people in this crazy health and fitness industry are capitalizing off of their luck and gene pool. I, on the other hand, fight with my gene pool every day. I swim in my pool of tears, battling my body's ability to process insulin. I do not eat the cake at parties because I cannot get away with it.

My battle is real. My battle is sometimes all-encompassing. My true fight is to harness this flame and put it towards good, or it will burn me alive. That is the naked truth behind my obsessive research, experiment, and scribbled discoveries.

This is a story I am still writing. I know that my journey with autoimmunity, insulin, inflammation, and a healthy gut is ongoing. I am reminded of this every time my hormones act up in the face of an indulgent weekend, and the PCOS acne says, "Hey, girl, heyyyyy!" Or after a few weeks of just eating a little more sugar here and there I put on ten pounds like nobody's business.

This is real. This is not me being one of those girls who needs to lose three pounds. This is me playing the hand I was dealt, trying to wear a smile behind my haute pink lipstick.

So that is who the fuck I am to write a book—a bitch who has gone through a lot, hit the floor hard a few times, and finally found a way to make it right and dance back on top of the table. I repeat, I am not a nutritionist. I am simply a life hacker who got lucky and finally found what works for my body and my health. Take my thoughts for what they are worth and find what works best for you and YOUR body.

I hope my message is simple. I hope you laugh. And I hope you learn to love your body in a way I never thought I could. Even you, Jessica.

X to the ohh Whitters

EAT.

You mustn't be afraid to eat a little more butter, darling.

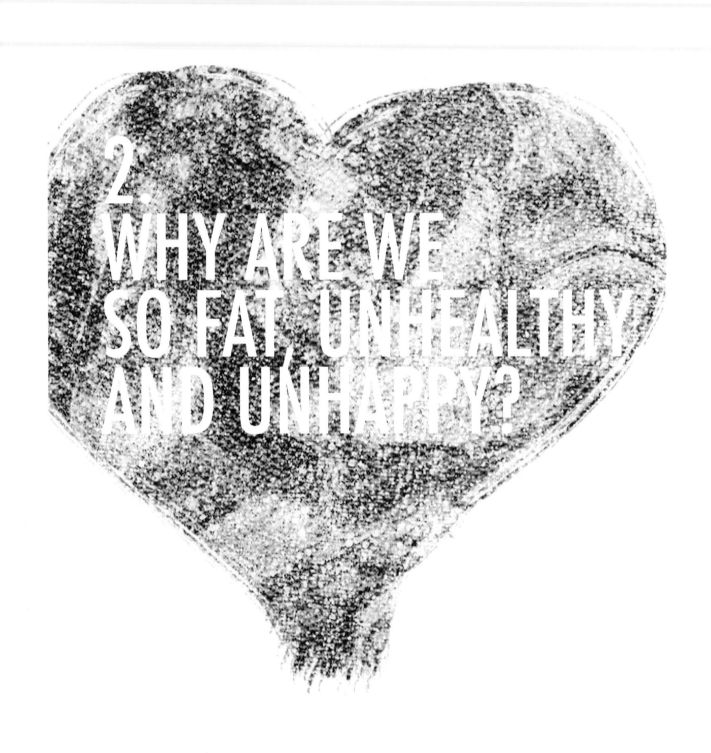

2.
WHY ARE WE SO FAT, UNHEALTHY AND UNHAPPY?

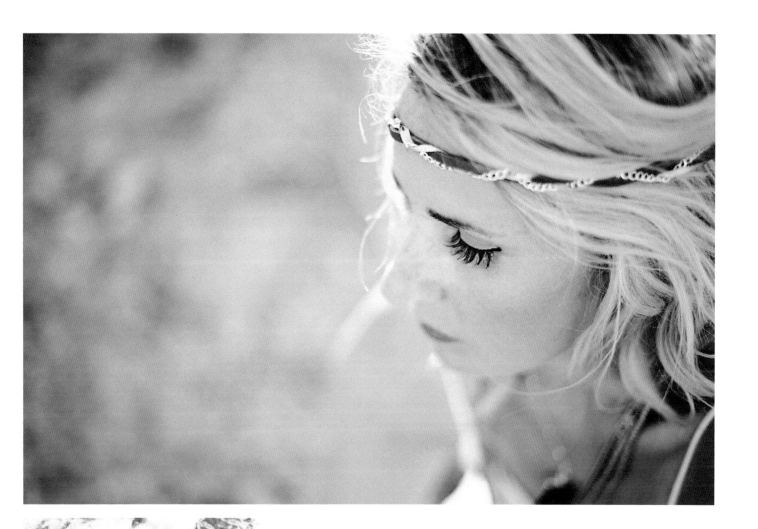

2. Why are we so fat, unhealthy, and unhappy?

Whip out your violin as I start by singing my sad, sad song on why I am easily made fat, unhealthy, and unhappy. As you may have already gathered, my body has a difficult time with insulin.

Insulin helps control blood glucose levels by signaling the liver, muscles and fat cells to take in glucose from the blood. So it helps with everything from energy, to fat loss, to hormone regulation.

I developed insulin resistance and either as a result or precursor, developed conditions where my body attacks itself.

Autoimmunity is my curse, and I unfortunately learned this the hard way through multiple diagnoses, prescriptions, tears, and anger.

Although I like to say that I beat disease and infertility, my body may never use insulin as effectively or easily as it was born to. My body may never unlearn how to attack itself.

I know this because in just a few days of eating too much sugar or too many carbs, my body flares up. My flares come in the form of retaining water, achy joints, acne, and cramping. I know right away when insulin is pissed at me, and I immediately back off the carbs and up the ante in fat and protein.

If my body reacted to insulin as it should, I would not have developed rheumatoid arthritis (RA) or polycystic ovarian syndrome (PCOS), both of which are my body's reaction to a problem, and not separate, unrelated unfortunate incidences.

Or maybe it is actually my fault. If I had fed my body foods that actually resembled some sort of digestible nutrient instead of the constant surge of glucose, I would not have put my body into a constant state of inflammation, I would not have developed insulin resistance, and I would not have developed RA or PCOS.

Because in the state of too much sugar your body stops regulating hormones the way it should, it stops detoxifying the way it should and in short, it tries to clean up the glucose driven inflammation by attacking itself.

This is why I believe that those who suffer from similar insulin, inflammation, and autoimmune driven conditions can, and will, feel better if they reduce their intake of refined carbs, processed anything, and sugar. You may need to do much, much more, but there is hope.

I know, I know, a correlation does not mean causation. But that does not mean that my anecdotal evidence is wrong.

So that is why you suck at life, now tell me why we are all so chunky and cranky?

Short answer: We left nature and found sugar.

You can take my anecdotal evidence for what it is, but most Americans want, but more so, need to feel better. Most Americans simply need to find some nature and ditch some sugar to feel better.

Most Americans make the same mistakes I did as a child and young adult. We were never taught what or how to eat; we were just taught to eat and then starve ourselves when we felt chunky.

Do you ever feel like you are doing everything right but are still just kind of chubby?

Why is it so easy to gain weight but so difficult to lose it?

Why is being and staying healthy so confusing?

Should this be simpler?

It should.

Think of plants and wild animals. Plants need things like water and nutrient rich soil. Animals need to hunt and forage from the land. They need sleep. They need water. They do not have an obesity epidemic… Well house pets do, but not animals in the wild…

You know from kindergarten that all of these things in the plant and animal kingdom are true. Why is that so easy to understand, but then we look at us humans and think, *thaa fuck happened there?*

This is the part of the story where I preach, sister, preach.

We left the animal kingdom. We left nature. We left the cave (though I promise not to talk about how we need to be cavemen. Please believe this bitch right here needs her lipstick, her deodorant, and her selfie a day iPhone.).

We stopped eating real plants and healthy animals. We stole animals from their nature, so they stopped eating real plants and other healthy animals. We effectively stole their health (and happiness) too.
We traded whole foods for w(hole-in-your-gut) grains.

We gnaw on diet food bars, inhale organic-non-fat-whole-grain everything, count every calorie, and here we still are—chubby and hangry. In a sentence, we are fat because of sugar, no longer cooking, no longer enjoying food, microwaving everything, factory farming, working too much, and sleeping too little. Oh, and sugar.

We have been practicing unsafe science and have built a food system that is extremely profitable at the pricey cost of our digestibility, and then our health. We have replaced the comfort of mealtime with the ease of convenience.

Our foods are overly processed, full of chemicals and added sugars, and our bodies simply don't know where to put this crap.

We are chronically dehydrated, and we are starving. Yes. The fattest country in the world is starving.

Eating fat-free pretty packages disguised as food and having more body fat than lean muscle tissue in the age of cardio, cardio, cardio has basically evolved us to be fat storing machines! Our cells are unable to function properly and seriously think we are starving because they never get the nutrients they need to survive, let alone thrive.

Without good fats, proteins, and essential nutrients, our bodies adapted from the caveman days to store our food as fat to survive a looming famine. However, if you look at our donks, clearly we isn't starving. Because of this, we have no idea how to read our hunger and metabolic signals for what they truly need.

Ah, sugar, sugar.

We are literally addicted to sugar because it is the only thing we have taught our bodies to use for energy in the modern age of whole grains washed down with 5-Hour Energy.

It has been said that we now consume **upwards of 400%** more sugar than we did in the 70's. Our genetic makeup tells us that anything sweet is safe to eat and not poisonous, so the addiction runs deep.

Bastards of evolution! Craving sugar is in my genes, so I'm gonna go ahead and crush this non-fat decaf carmel frappawhata with Splenda flooded sugar-free caramel syrup, but hold the whip! I is on a diet!

I do not want to get into the artificial sweetener debate, but in my opinion it is made from chemicals and just perpetuates our addiction to something sweet, like more sugar from more carbs.

I think anything with sugar-free or fat-free on the label actually should read, *promotes fat storage and potentially cancer.*

But like I said, I ain't going there, not today.

It is this simple: evolution has programmed our bodies to crave things that will not get us killed and will promote our thriving survival.

We think we crave sugar, but we actually crave a way of life that feeds our bodies nutrients, FAT and foods we are able to digest and use for energy.

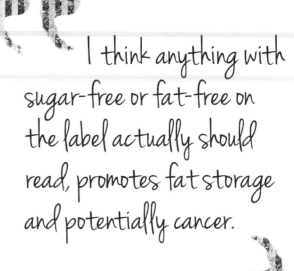

I think anything with sugar-free or fat-free on the label actually should read, promotes fat storage and potentially cancer.

NERD SUGAR: Glycogen and Insulin

Your liver performs many essential functions related to digestion, metabolism, immunity, and the storage of nutrients within the body. So from that we can go ahead and assume it is imperative to your health and survival.

Another function of your liver is to convert glucose (sugar/carbs) to glycogen to store and use for energy. It cannot store that much glycogen, so the rest has to be stored in muscle tissue. But, we eat so many carbs and foods made in a lab that our livers are overworking, confused, and starting to break down.

Muscle tissue has a very small capacity to store glycogen. We also tend to have much less muscle tissue than our primal uncles, so our glycogen ends up spilling into our bloodstream. Insulin tries to shove the glucose into our muscles and bloodstream anyway. But it just won't zip, so it enters our fat cells, which are roomy!

Insulin is supposed to regulate blood sugar and ensure the delivery of nutrients throughout your body. But when insulin levels rise due to excess glucose, insulin can no longer focus on delivering nutrients because it's dealing with the sewage of a blood stream you've dealt it.

This precious gift of higher insulin makes us think we are hungry, so we eat more shit. This is bad news for our abs (and our overall health, but let's be honest we just wanna look good naked).

Once your body is no longer sensitive to insulin, a dangerous chain of events occurs. Excessive inflammation forms in your body, sometimes triggering your body to attack its own tissue, as is the case in autoimmune conditions.

Insulin stops supplying glycogen (energy) to lean muscle tissue, so your body takes everything it consumes for quick energy and then sends everything else to fat storage. Among other faults in your metabolism, your liver, insulin, and bloodstream are not delivering nutrients. Your body thinks you are starving.

Your good old liver slowly becomes covered in fat unable to transport nutrients to the body, dispel toxins, give us energy, or help our body fight infection and disease. This is the point where you should be more concerned about your health and less about your abs.

Do you ever wonder why people who are non-drinkers seem to have intense liver issues? Too much sugar broken down from too many carbs breaks the system, leading to insulin resistance, which leads to excessive inflammation, diabetes, and organ failure to be blunt.

Digestion: The New Diet Pill

Do you ever wonder what happens after that bite? That food has a few options. It can be used for immediate energy. It can be stored as fat. Or it can feed the good, and, unfortunately, the bad bacteria in your gut. Your body's ultimate goal is energy usage and cellular nourishment. When these two primal needs are not met, the food we eat promotes fat storage and inflammation.

Digestion. *Cell food. Body fuel. Improper digestion.*

Cell starvation. *Body screaming for fuel. You feeling ravenous after a huge bowl of whole grain cereal.*

I'd argue that too many low quality carbohydrates and the lack of quality fat and nutrients is not only making us fat, it is killing us. Every carbohydrate you put in your mouth, be it fruit, organic cheddar bunnies, or a healthy non-fat yogurt with low-fat granola and honey, breaks down to sugar in your body (glucose converted to glycogen for energy if we are getting nerdy).

What your body cannot breakdown—WHICH is a lot—is stored in fat cells. AND/or it becomes food for intestinal bacteria leading to a host of issues such as inflammation and chronic diseases. Hello, rheumatoid arthritis (RA) and polycystic ovarian syndrome (PCOS)! My name is Whitney!

Wonders of science like high-fructose corn syrup and vegetable oils were only made available in the last one hundred years but are now found in almost anything edible in a package.

Today, more people get cancer, heart disease, are fatter, more diabetic, and are ridden with chronic conditions like arthritis and skin disorders than people living one-hundred years ago. We may live longer these days, but we are not, in my opinion, healthier.

Nor are we *really* living. We should just feel alive, move freely, and enjoy each day, but our diagnoses seem to get the best of many of us.

Fact. We are not digesting "our food." That is why we are fat. That is why we are sick. That is why we are so unhappy and constantly hungry.

Fact. The way *you* can process and digest food is totally different than the way *I* can. That means you have to sort out what your body can use for fuel and what it cannot. Annoying, I know.

Make sense so far?

Bonus:

Watch this Ted Med talk by one of my idols, Dr. Peter Attia, who discusses insulin resistance and the obesity epidemic.

NERD NOTES:

Eating less carbs (sugar) + nutrients to all cells + not sending body into false starvation + insulin in check + healthy liver

=

Someday seeing your ABS!! (again or for the first time)

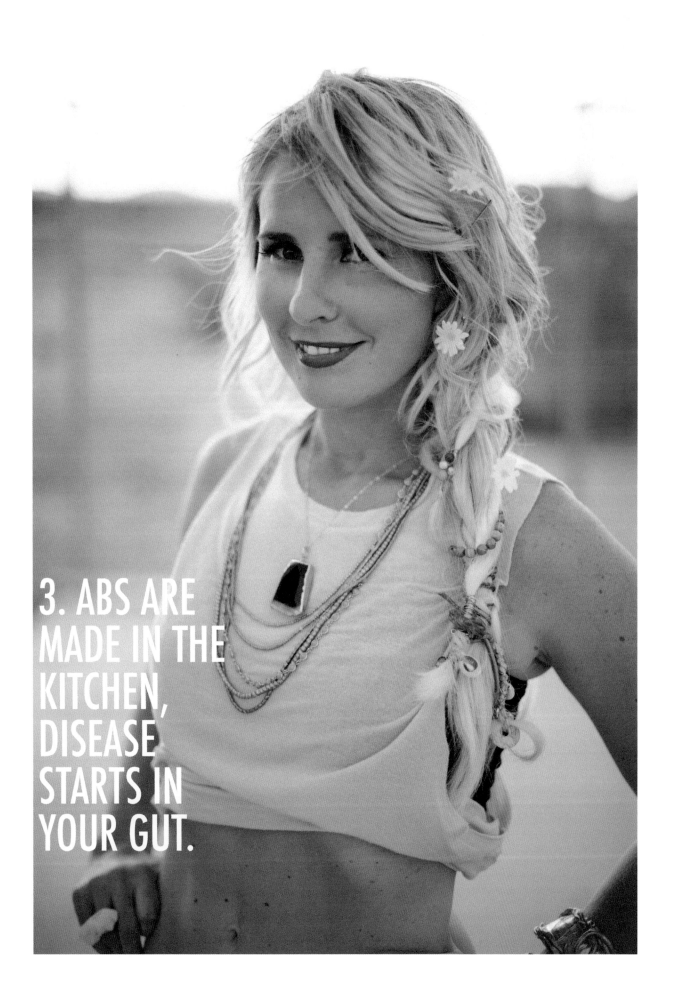

3. ABS ARE MADE IN THE KITCHEN, DISEASE STARTS IN YOUR GUT.

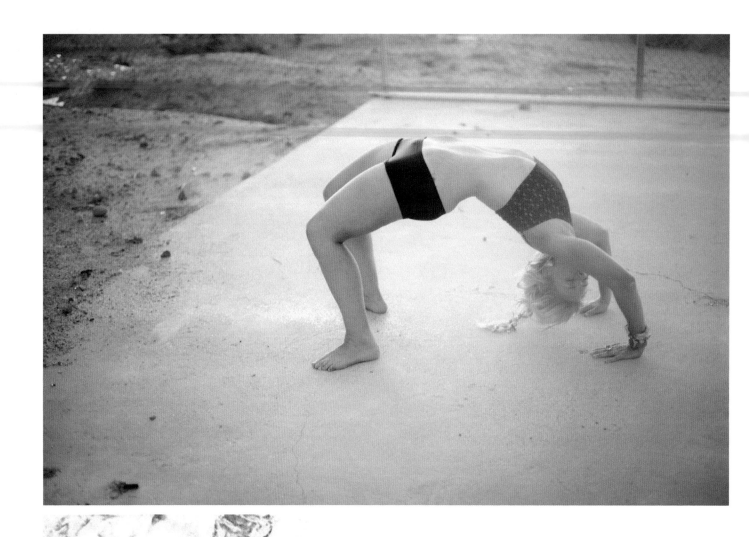

3. ABS ARE MADE IN THE KITCHEN, DISEASE STARTS IN YOUR GUT.

"All disease begins in the gut."
-Hippocrates

Read and memorize this thousand-year-old quote. Go ahead read it again. And again. And again. And one more time.

The biggest mistake I made from the day I started tearing out shreds of skinny models and plastering them around my room was damaging the lining of my gut looking for the magic bullet to look like those models.

What would get me the thinnest the fastest?

Diet pills at fourteen? Yep I tried that. Diet Rockstars and protein bars? Boom let's do this.

Synthetic who knows what kind of hormones you buy on the internet from who knows who? Oh yeah, let's go ahead and soak in that goodness.

Starve yourself and then gorge on cheat day? That one was my personal fave. Looking for tips in heartbreaking "Ana's Girls" forums and wearing a rubber band around my wrist to snap myself when I felt hungry?

Yes, and it hurts admitting it. It hurts real deep.

"Ana's Girls" is, unfortunately, a secret group of girls identifying themselves online in forums and chat rooms to support each other in the practice of anorexia. Yep, I feel your heart breaking.

Every new diet, fad, or trend I tried was just a little more harsh on my gut, organs, and soul. It is amazing how intelligent your gut actually is.

If it aches, if it constantly feels bloated, if you cannot poop, if you get upset stomach frequently, your gut is trying to smack you across the face and wake you up.

I remember in and out of all the crap I put my body through how terribly my stomach would ache, how I would get headaches every day, and how puffy my entire body would be.

My gut even told me one day that I needed to eat meat again. Thank God I started to listen to what it had to say.

I believe with my whole heart that the impetus for developing rheumatoid arthritis (RA) and polycystic ovarian syndrome (PCOS) was my unhealthy gut married to an abusive mind. If I had focused on healing my gut and my head from the first moment my joints ached, I would have saved myself years of pain and heartache.

My gut lining had simply become so damaged that I was not absorbing (or even consuming) the nutrients and enzymes I needed. Insulin ran rampant, and my body literally started to attack itself as remnants of food, toxins, and bad bacteria found their way into my bloodstream and who knows where else. I was inflamed, in pain, chubby, and depressed.

Every specialist I saw gave me more pills, potentially furthering the disease by irritating my gut with ingredients that harm good bacteria.

I was given meds such as NSAIDs (non-steroidal anti-inflammatory drug) and antibiotics. Not one doctor asked me what my diet looked like. Not one. But every last one of them knew I needed another magic pill.

Living in the moment of diagnosis, you trust your doctors because you are so desperate to feel better and simply do not have the knowledge to challenge the system.

Looking back, you feel angry. Are they trying to keep a secret from you? The secret that gut health may actually be both the cause and the cure.

Feel free to sit and let the juices marinate on that last one. Yes, what I am saying is that all of your problems could very well be a result of your unhealthy gut.

Gut health: The Real Magic Bullet to Health and Abs

A healthy gut sets the stage for good nutrient absorption, a healthy immune system, reduced inflammation, and a strong metabolism.

Your metabolism (starting in the gut) not only decides how good you look naked, it more importantly determines your body's ability to fight infection and disease.

So if your intestinal lining is diet soda soaked and trying to break down all the healthy protein bars you bathe in, we have a problem.

Fact. Gut health is the most important factor in your metabolism and your immune system. They say 80% of your health stems from your gut, so thriving digestion and absorption through your gut is the secret to the abs and happiness you have always wanted ([1]).

Fact. Your gut is the front line of your immune system, housing good bacteria marines and fighting bad bacteria militants. Its job is to make sure only fully digested particles pass through the intestinal wall, and to protect against toxins, bad bacteria, and waste before it enters the rest of the body. However, we tend to eat so many food irritants like wheat, sugar, Cheez-its, sugar, canola oil, sugar, and whole grains that over time tiny gaps form in our gut.

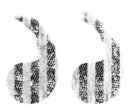

The secret that gut health may actually be both the cause and the cure.

Tiny gaps in your gut, aka leaky gut syndrome, allow undigested food particles, more toxins, and waste to enter your blood stream. This causes all kinds of ruckus like inflammation, insulin resistance, hormonal disruption, and eventually autoimmune disease as our bodies cannot discriminate between our own tissue and the "food" we feed it.

This is a simplified but truthful explanation:

Poor gut health = poor immune health = inflammation = chub rub = opening the door for disease.

I highly encourage you to study gut health on your own and look into your own personal gut function. You would be amazed and so lucky to realize how many problems can be healed or reversed simply by focusing on your gut.

If you desire any of the following, it's time for a gut check.

- Look good naked
- Avoid getting sick
- Avoid developing disease
- Have optimal hormonal function for great skin and to get preggers (someday)
- Better moods

Heal Thy Gut, Heal Thyself

Hopefully at this point in our story, you are concerned about your own gut health. You realize that you have to get to a place where you no longer want the quickest route to a beach bod; you want the best route to a healthy gut, which may in time get you that beach bod after all.

You have to observe how foods and supplements make you feel. Feel good. Look good. When foods digest properly, you will feel better in your own skin, in every sense of the word.

There is Hope

Please know, if you are struggling with any hormonal issue, chronic disease, and potentially infertility, my heart sits with yours. I do believe there is hope.

I do believe you should stop reading this immediately and book an appointment with a respected naturopathic doctor in your area. Yes, it will be expensive. No, insurance may not cover it. It will be worth it in the end. If you cannot afford it and/or are too afraid to try, please do your best to HEAL your gut on your own.

I will get into a good three-week approach to nourishing a healthy gut later, but if you are seriously concerned about your own gut health or have any type of hormonal dysfunction or autoimmune conditions, I challenge you to don your white coat and start researching.

Look for studies, readings, and recipes on the following:
- Autoimmune protocol
- Autoimmune disease and gut health
- Gut health
- Leaky gut
- GAPS Diet
- Autoimmune diet
- Heal leaky gut with food

What It All Means to Me

In avoiding grains, junky meat, excess sugar, and processed foods, I reduced and eliminated the RA. By eating more healthy animals, more vegetables, and very little carbs I kicked PCOS out of the way and got myself KNOCKED up.

I believe I did what a naturopathic doctor would have told me to do—remove all irritating foods (eliminate grains, sugar, overly processed cheap meats), renourish (consume more nutrients from veggies and good organic pasture-raised meats), repopulate good gut bacteria (daily probiotics and prebiotics from yogurt, sauerkraut, and pickles, oh my!).

Instead of taking the advice of a naturopath, I took the route of listening to my body, which I do not entirely recommend because it was painful and took years. My advice to you is to have a real gut check and heart-to-heart with yourself.

Is your gut as healthy as it should be? Did you try something for a little while and abandon the path because you didn't see results over night?

Ask and answer yourself honestly, and then get to work. If you truly want to heal, you need to be willing to invest months, possibly even years into this work on yourself.

GUT CHECK: The Research

Fact. The lining of your gut needs to be damaged in order for autoimmune diseases to develop (study here).

"Autoimmune" basically means the immune system is acting against itself, potentially punishing you for feeding it shit it cannot breakdown or use for nutrients, though the second part of that statement is only my theory.

Fact. Autoimmune diseases can be improved and even reversed by REPAIRING the damage to your gut (2.). Real life proof? Me, 1. rheumatoid arthritis, 0.

Fact. If your gut is compromised, you are not digesting all of your food, and not soaking in the nutrients you need for proper hormonal and enzymatic function (3). Think infertility and thyroid troubles. Real life proof? Me again!

My good friend polycystic ovarian syndrome has left the building, and my one-year-old is napping soundly in his crib (hopefully for another hour).

Fact. Foods that irritate my gut the most are grains, junky dairy, and sugar. Source = instant pain and swelling in my hands and feet, bloated tummy, chub, and years of infertility.

BONUS READ: Get Knocked Up!

Considering the Rice Krispies and Diet everything I was bathing in for years, it is truly my belief that I severely damaged my gut lining and function (leaky gut syndrome), which then developed into autoimmune dysfunction (RA), disrupted hormone function, and compromised my fertility (PCOS). Phew, that there was a mouthful!

This study reports that PCOS is actually caused by disturbances in good gut flora, and another study suggests that infertility and pregnancy loss can largely be caused by autoimmunity (your immune system attacking its own tissue).

Simply put, 80% of our immune system LIVES in our gut so if it is leaking, allowing bad bacteria in, and unable to remove toxins, our bodies will basically protect themselves from getting pregnant because the immune system is too busy and/or compromised to protect and nourish a growing fetus.

In nerd speak, here is what scientists and doctors believe is happening to Fertile Myrtle. First, if autoantibodies show up to the party because our body is dealing with leftover food particles (toxins and pathogens otherwise taken care of by a strong gut), infertility occurs regardless if your body has developed an autoimmune disease. The presence of autoantibodies basically means your body is starting to attack itself.

Second, autoimmunity may affect all stages of fertility, via ovarian failure, testicular failure in men, implantation failure, and pregnancy loss. Third, infertility may also be secondary to vasculitis (inflammation in the blood vessels) associated with other conditions such as lupus and diabetes (4).

Basically (and I am OVERSIMPLIFYING here), leaky gut starts happening, then inflammation starts forming in your lining and blood stream, triggering the autoantibodies to surface, damaging your immune system and blocking your body's ability to conceive and protect a growing child.

Need more? Nutrients and minerals affect hormones. If your gut lining is damaged, your body's ability to absorb nutrients and minerals diminishes, and hormones have to be in balance for conception to occur.

Finally, most leaky gut victims have a challenge with excessive yeast, which terrorizes the reproductive organs by causing not only intestinal inflammation but also poisons you with the by-products of the yeast.

In short, an unhealthy gut creates a toxic environment within your body potentially blocking your ability to conceive (5.). I totally can feel this through a PCOS flare up of bloating and cranky cramping!

What we can conclude is this: bad gut health results in an imbalanced immune system and very whacky hormones, which may attack your body's ability to get pregnant.

NERD NOTES:

- Gut health = barefoot and pregnant, six pack abs, immune health
- Heal your gut lining and repopulate good gut bacteria = reduce inflammation = potential reversal/suppression of autoimmune conditions!
- Gut health = the magic bullet

4. MEN ARE STUPID

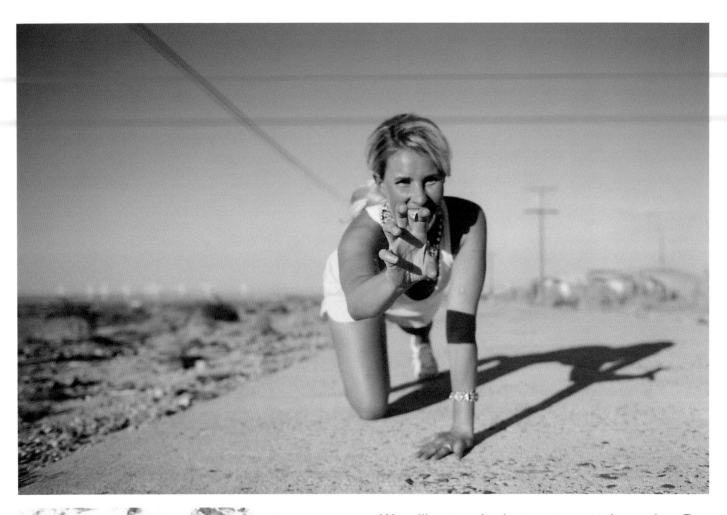

4. Men are Stupid.

Why do women seem to have more fat, and why is it so easy for men to lose weight?

- Short answer = Muscle mass.
- Testosterone. Child bearing.
- Choosing the elliptical machine over strength training.
- Evil seventh grade girls.

We will get to the last statement, I promise. But first I need you to understand a thing or two about muscle and our ability to turn food into energy or storage on our hips.

Lesson 1

Muscle stores glycogen (carbs) for energy to be used as needed.

Lesson 2

We beezies have less muscle than men, so our blessed ability to store carbs (glycogen) as fat is, quite frankly, aggressive.

Conclusion

Because women have less muscle tissue, we have more room on our hips for fat.
And some more bullshit, our good friend estrogen helps us store fat, whereas men have testosterone, which burns fat. Holler for a dollar, honey boo boo!

We also have the babies.

Our bodies have the ability to carry children and again caveman shit—we store fat for our survival and that of our pending offspring. That is just what it is, and if you're preggers, that first trimester is game over for not having carbs. I showered in Smart Puffs, Pop Chips, and ginger candies.

Useless note:

My super scientific guess is that my body probably craved carbs because my ancestors told me they could be stored as fat in case famine hit, so my child would survive. Not to mention opening the fridge made me want to barf so the action of cooking was pretty much out, leaving my pregnant self hungry for nutrients.

Luckily, I went back to low sugar, more fat, and no grains after the first trimester. I had a very healthy pregnancy, little weight gain, and pissed a lot of glitter in those cups at the doctor's offce. But that's another story, for another time.

Evil Seventh Grade Girls and Emotionally Induced Chub

I am going to go out on a limb and say one of the reasons women are "fatter" than men is because we are meaner to each other and biologically more emotional.

I know! I know! I just gone and sent us way back a few decades, but we are. You know it. I know it.
We just have more feelings, okay!

We judge each other in bikinis, in the locker room, and at the grocery store. We are so insecure in our own skin that we have tried EVERYTHING to look better for our frienemies.

Our "trying" always comes at an irrational decision-making moment and always ends in some sort of crash and burn. Stay with me on this. In fact, take your crazy for a walk with mine.

If you look back to the times you dieted or sought the comfort of consumption, what was the trigger?

For me, the first "love" of my life broke my heart = anorexia.

Working out a ton, lifting a ton, playing softball five hours a day, and being diagnosed with rheumatoid arthritis as a collegiate athlete = overeating pothead.

Doctor said I couldn't get pregnant = alcoholic.

Every terrible diet turn for me has stemmed from emotion until I made myself miserable enough to make a change.

We consume from emotion.

Peer pressure, combined with the tough shit that happens in our life, has set us up to seek very quick fixes for our bodies. Every time, we wreak havoc on our metabolism and overall health, both physically and emotionally.

In some instances like starving ourselves, we are rewarded with rapid weight loss. We always remember that "success" and have trouble remembering that we gained ALL of the weight back and then some in the short weeks after.

Through this destruction, we lose pounds but not true fat. We never build the muscle tissue needed to keep the weight off, and we destroy our metabolism in the process.

Our greatest motivator is fat loss, but we just seem to be losing weight and self-esteem. We aggressively gain weight alongside the self-inflicting behavior of emotional eating.

I do not just mean eating chocolate because you are depressed, I mean not eating or torturing yourself over inches, calories, and numbers on a scale that engulfs our being. We are so consumed by numbers that we are never able to see the strength in our bodies and lead ourselves blindly into a life of *counting cardio*. Count calories in, watch the numbers on the treadmill burn them; rinse and repeat for a miserable lifetime.

I personally have weighed myself at the gym, only to cry the whole drive home over five maybe ten pounds.

Nowadays, I find a happy balance in weighing myself every two weeks, no more no less. This keeps me on track and prevents a mess of a meltdown on my hub's shoulders. I am human, and a girl; sorry about that.

Start Serving Love

Fact. Being nicer to each other and ourselves will change your body. Greater fact. Selecting your tribe is very important as they will nourish or harm you in a significantly greater capacity than food ever will. This is the honest and humbling truth.

My body really made the most changes when I started appreciating it for all that it can do—like play sports well and harvest a small child.

My friend, January, played a tremendous role in my soul search for nourishment and self love. She helped me realize that you cannot have a nourished body without a nourished soul, meaning you have to love yourself to truly take care of yourself.

Without her, this book does not exist. I'd like to think we continue to teach each other about patience, acceptance, and speaking your truth in all aspects of your life.

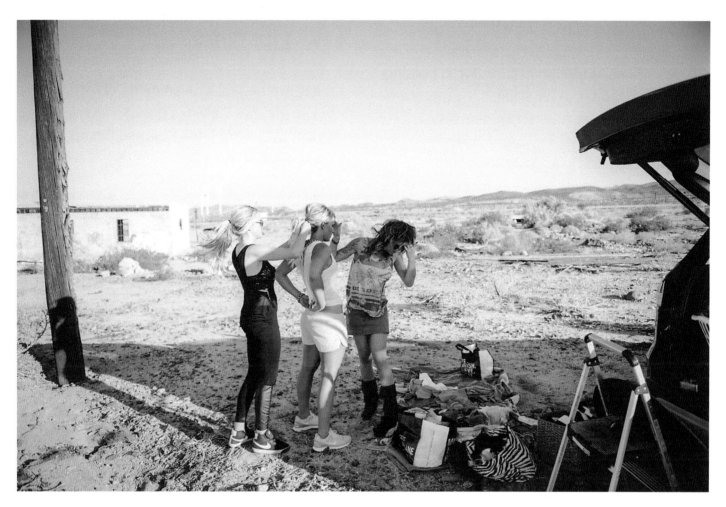

Surrounding yourself with great people makes you greater.

Trim the fat with friends and family who do not nourish your soul. My friends and family make fun of the way I eat on the reg (regular for us not so hip folk); however, they do so in a loving, curious way.

I am not saying to blow off anyone who questions why all the sudden there is butter in your coffee. I am saying make a conscious decision to surround yourself with individuals that make you better, a coven that makes each other stronger.

Fact. When you have babies, it really does take a village, so start trading in favors and love now. I thank the stars for my sister wives, Savannah and Brittany, and my ridiculously amazing and selfless mother.
Without them, my life is a hot mess and not the good kind of haute.

One of the most difficult things you have to do in life is consciously choose to avoid people who are toxic. You may love them deep in your bones, but there will be times you have to step away from them to focus on your own health and that of your loved ones. This is not selfish. This is you protecting your own fragile mental health.

You do not have to breakup with your BFF; but if she is in a self-inflicting cycle of pain and abuse, you have tried to help and ain't nothing gonna help, you may have to just quietly stop reaching out to her and let her deal a bit.

Misery really does love company, and sometimes the healthiest thing for both of you is to walk away for a bit and inspire her with your own happiness. You will find relationships change, evolve, and even end depending on where you are in your life and mental health. This is okay. Breathe through it.

While I realize we are getting into some hippie territory here, it is truth. Learn to love other women for who they are, what they can teach us, and the bodies they house. Learn to appreciate the body and soul you house, because loving means taking care of you. You will learn to appreciate our differences, our curves, our stems, and our donks.

Coat your day in nourishment, love, and truth, and I promise you will find happiness and the abs you really dream of.

This means we have to start calling each other out on our bullshit self-deprecating banter. Tell your friends the following, "If you ask me if I can see your fat, my new rule is to bitch slap it!" Don't join her pity party. The biggest way to influence change in others is to be an aspiring change that DOES NOT preach at them.

I am guilty of preaching from time to time and always have the best results with others by keeping my mouth shut and applying love.

Love Your Booty.

I'd say for the first two-ish thirds of my life, I did not like my butt. I always got attention for it. Boys like it (I think), but I felt like it made me look so weird.

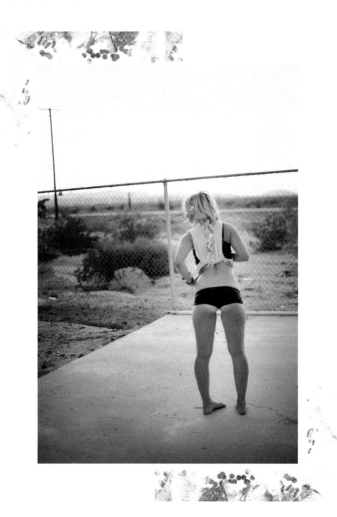

To this day, clothes can be a struggle because things just do not fit well with a donk. Dresses do not lay right. Shorts do not button. You go bare ass every time you sit down in jeans. You been there? Holler.

Butt now, I embrace it. I dare say I love my butt. As women, we are subconsciously taught not to take well to compliments about our body, and as a result we find ways of also not loving our bodies.

Butt, we have to love our bodies, for they are the only place we have to live; if we are not kind to our bodies, they will not last long. And/or we will be miserable for life, and what kind of life is that?

I got it from my momma. I love her butt; I always have. I loved slapping it as a kid. Even now, nothing gives me greater joy than a good donk grab/slap for my mommy.

So here is my donk world. She is big. She gives me bu-thigh lines. She has cellulite. She's the last one to leave a party. And goddammit, she's here for a good time.

Love your booty. Love your body.

Science to Go Along with Our Warm Cup of Misery

Now that we are holding hands, let's go ahead and end our honeymoon.

Every time we miss a meal or cut calories—every single time—our bodies release fat storing lipogenic enzymes.

These nasty little boogers are trying to make sure we don't starve, so along the way they help us destroy our wonderful fat burning lipolytic enzymes. And, of course, God's gift to women was to make sure this has a more profound effect on us than it does on men (6).

If I had to guess, I would say the history of "starve yourself until 6 p.m. diets" most women (have attempted) effected the actual study results. Meaning the women they studied had already conditioned their bodies to need the fat storing enzymes after years of terrible dieting, enzymatic and hormonal abuse.

Fact. You have to eat to keep your hormones, enzymes, and metabolism working optimally well together. Your metabolism, hormonal function, and enzymatic output may serve different needs and purposes within your body, but they are all interconnected.

If enzymes and hormones are not functioning properly, neither will your metabolism. When enzymatic activity is disrupted or missing the nutrients needed to function, overactive and under active hormonal situations (such as overactive and under active thyroid) start to occur (7.).

Cheating on the Treadmill: The Bulky Truth

Fact. Cardio will not make you healthier; muscle will. I could argue that muscle is arguably the most physically important component of our metabolism.

The amount of muscle you have determines your resting metabolic rate, which in a nutshell is the amount of energy you burn when you is just parked on the couch doing big things. If you have more muscle, you burn more calories, allowing you to eat and cheat a bit more! Yum.

Now most trainers will tell you that women cannot "bulk" up. We don't have the testosterone to build muscle like men, and to them I say horse shit. Even though they are technically right and serve you good intentions, what is wrong is our diet and need for chronic cardio **on top** of a strength training program that causes us to **look** bulky.

Not only are we building muscle which increases in size, we are not burning the fat stored underneath it fast enough; seeing is believing, buttercup.

Though you may actually be building beautiful muscle tissue and well on your way to improving your metabolism and your bod, we quit the minute we look and feel bigger.

I still have these moments where I am making serious muscle gains. But suddenly, my shorts are tighter, and I just want to cry and abandon my strength routine.

Stick through the bulk and your routine for a few more weeks. If anything, check your diet first, and your strength routine if, and only if, you do not see the changes in your body you are looking for.

Start asking these questions when you "feel" bulky and want a plea bargain with the treadmill.

Are you resting enough?

Fat storing happens when you are not sleeping or resting well.

Is your body inflamed because you are overworking your muscles?

Never allowing your muscles to recover inhibits their growth and change AND it helps you store fat, because your body thinks you are stressed.

Are you giving your body the nutrients it needs with increased muscle?

Without nutrients, your body will store fat, despite your hard work.

Are you consuming too much sugar from healthy shakes and fruit?

Super easy mistake to make, just because it is "healthy," we tend to overeat it.

Muscles and Munchies

Now muscle creates more energy demands in our bods, which reveals itself as big time hunger. Instead of nourishing muscle tissue with good fats and proteins from clean meats or digestible good carbs like sweet potatoes, we feed our body shit wrapped in a package deemed healthy because it is under 150 calories from a list of about 35 ingredients.

Or we are showering in whole grains believing we NEED the carbs and fiber! We are unable to fully digest them or use them for energy and are missing nutrients our new muscle craves.

So, our hunger signals tell us to keep on eating, creating a vicious cycle of wanting to quit our new strength routine and return to a life on the treadmill fueled by the 100 calorie menu. It is easy to abandon ship at this point. You can see in the mirror that you are not burning fat because you are not physically smaller.

Peace out, starving myself it is!

And never giving your body a chance to adjust and prosper for a lifetime.

Men Are Stupid.

Men who start a weight training program are at an advantage because they have more muscle tissue and testosterone on their side to build more healthy muscle tissue. This makes them inherently better and faster at burning fat than women.

Their bodies are simply more efficient at using the garbage they eat for energy. When we think it is easier for them, it really is. Not to mention, for the most part, they want to get bigger, so muscle gains keep them mentally in the game when us beezies gone ahead and checked out! Abandoning, or never adopting a strength routine, is hands down one of the biggest mistakes women make in their journey to a better body.

Build lean muscle tissue, eat well, and stay lean for life. Build a little tiny bit of muscle tissue on the elliptical, eat protein bars, and stay soft wondering why you always feel bloated for life.

We will get into the specifics of muscles and how to rock 'em in chapter nine. For now, start treating muscle as part of your metabolism.

Let's Recap, Love Child.

Eat better, not less. Stop giving a shit what others think. Love other women. Do less cardio. Add more muscle. Look better naked. Sounds too easy right?

Fact. The damage you have done to your entire system, physically and mentally, may take some time to heal. But it should be clear that if you would like to be fit for a lifetime, you have to start nourishing yourself for a lifetime. You have to consume good calories that will feed your body the nutrients and enzymes needed to thrive.

Fact. Some days I fucking suck at life. I feel ugly, fat, bloated, and want to punch someone in the face. These days will always happen although for the most part I do love myself and on most days love my body. I am human; I am woman. My life will never be perfect, though I may try to outwardly show you that it is.

Fact. Eating a variety of good proteins and fats, fruits and vegetables, and the occasional delight will liberate your soul and your waistline. Having the "I don't give a shit what people think" attitude that men tend to have will help you make better choices and control emotional food triggers.

Say it straight; say it with a smile.

Find time for you, your loving coven, and health. It won't happen overnight, sweet cheeks, but with time you will nourish your way to the body and soul you love.

NERD NOTES:

More lean muscle + more nutrients + more
love + less carbs +
less cardio + strong coven
=
nourishing your body and soul = more energy
expenditure = proper hormonal and enzymatic
function = working metabolism = fat burn =
#smokinghautewife

5.
EAT FAT.

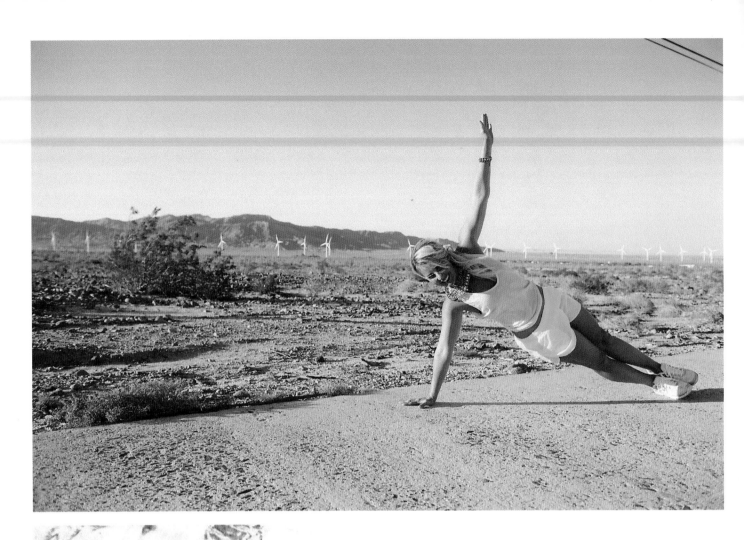

5. Eat. Fat.

"The body tends to be smarter than we think it is. Once you strip out all those processed foods that override your system and tend to make you overeat, your appetite becomes a great gauge of what you do."

— Dr. Peter Attia

You officially need to be really concerned with your body's response to insulin and way less concerned with cholesterol numbers. We have been obsessing over cholesterol numbers far too long, practicing unsafe science again without hearing cholesterol's side of the story.

I hear you singing and dancing while your bacon cooks in butter. Too much of a good thing is rarely that.

Anything in excess can create a toxic situation. A glass of wine—delightful. A bottle—headache.

Necessary fats and cholesterol, wonderful flow of hormones and bodily function. Too much fat combined with carbs you cannot breakdown. Your metabolism has no goddam idea what to do other than store that shit, and then allow it to wreak havoc on your intestinal lining, organs, and arteries.

Funny story. I drink coffee every day (earth shattering, I know). To which, I drink it one of two ways. Number one: I have a wonderful coffee shop (Caffe Calabria usually) make me a cappuccino.
Not just any shop, they have to know what they are doing. They have to roast their own beans or have an amazing supplier who does. My second option is at home served with butter, coconut oil, sea salt, and cinnamon. This is part of the reason I easily lost all the weight after pregnancy.

Everyone focuses on this buttery coffee. Everyone thinks, or simply wants to believe, that this was my magic bullet in weight loss. I get texts, emails, and Instagram messages asking for my recipe, and people desperate to know how butter in my coffee helped me lose weight.

This was one thing in a combination of many other things that helped me lose weight. If I drank this coffee and then downed a bowl of oatmeal, we would be singing a different tune.

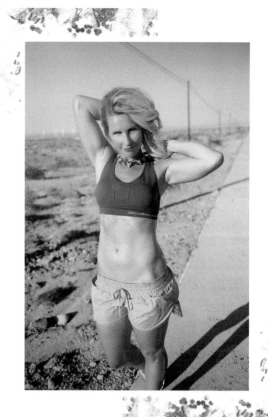

Fact. I lost all the pregnancy weight fairly easily because I was militant about what went in my body. I avoided sugar, grains, and drank limited amounts of alcohol for months. I ate good fats, proteins from healthy animals and a lot of greens. I drank a ton of water, walked everywhere I possibly could, and worked out slowly but surely.

It was more of a magic recipe than a bullet. It was a recipe to fuel my body with fat (ketones) instead of sugar (glucose). Otherwise known as a recipe of putting my body into a state of nutritional ketosis, which I will come back to later in our story.

This is NOT something I recommend doing over the long haul. Avoiding carbohydrates (or any macronutrient for that matter) can at some point mess with your hormones and digestion.

Buttered coffee will not help you if the rest of your day is full of carbs and sugar. In fact, it will likely hurt you. Too much sugar, or glucose broken down from carbs, makes typically good-for-you fats entirely too difficult to break down. Buttered coffee works for me because I consume a much lower amount of carbohydrates than most people.

We are getting a bit off topic here, but the point is this, consuming cholesterol is not the deadly bullet that is making you fat, ridden with disease, or struggling with hormonal imbalances.

You being unable to digest the foods you are eating, and/or the foods not serving any nutritional purpose is the cause you have to start fighting.

The Nerdy Deets

Fact. Cholesterol is needed in your body for life to continue to occur, and eating cholesterol has very little impact on the cholesterol levels in your body (8.). Whip out that bacon, my friend.

Fact. Cholesterol is actually a key building block for all cells and is produced by our bodies as a response to some sort of stress (9.). As a result, cholesterol is found in your body when it is trying to clean up after your party and then mistakenly gets blamed for the mess. When there is inflammation in your gut, cholesterol is needed to repair the gaps.

Sometimes the inflammation goes away as does the cholesterol. Unfortunately, most of the time, the inflammation gets worse so the cholesterol starts to oxidize and grow, taking up too much space in the artery, slowing the arterial flow, and causing clots.

Scientists blame cholesterol for clogging arteries and causing heart attacks when really cholesterol was just a symptom of the body trying to repair itself.

It's all one big fat unhealthy co-dependent relationship.

In health and chub there is no magic bullet. No one answer solves the equation for better or worse. It is ironic really. Things only become simple once you understand that the relationship between nutrition, disease, health, and metabolism is twisted and totally interconnected.
If nutrition, disease, and metabolism were to post their relationship status on Facebook, it would read: It's complicated, and we are unhealthily interdependent.

Everything is connected to everything else. Too many indigestible food particles and carbs cause inflammation, which can lead to cholesterol build up. And/or it can cause your body to no longer react to insulin, which can lead to hormonal trouble and significant fat storage. Or maybe it's in the reverse order? What came first—the chicken or the egg? All of these things affect one another directly or indirectly.

You simply cannot look at how cholesterol could be making you unhealthy; you have to step back and piece together the whole puzzle.

Are you digesting all of your food? Are you pooping? But really, are you? Are you eating a variety of nutrients? Are the nutrients you are eating actually being absorbed in the body because you have paired it with good fats, AND your gut is strong?
You absorb nutrients in your gut, you know. And . . .nutrients work best in the presence of other nutrients.

Similarly, enzymes and hormones in your body cannot function properly if one of those systems is broken. Do yourself a favor and stop wondering what the one thing is you should eat for the rest of your life to feel thin. Start eating real food from a variety of healthy animals and plants from the earth.

Bonus:

If you would like to read a scientific dissertation on all things cholesterol (first of all, awesome) I would kindly refer you to one of my idol's blogs, the Eating Academy by Dr. Peter Attia.

NERD NOTES:

- Poor digestion = Cholesterol build up. Hormones going wacky. Fat storage. Disease. Ruckus.
- Too much fat and/or carb consumption = fat gain.
- Fat + a lot of carbs = Fat gain.
- Fat + Greens + a litte carb = ABS

62. SO WHAT DO I EAT TO IS THIS GLITTER OU SPEAK F?

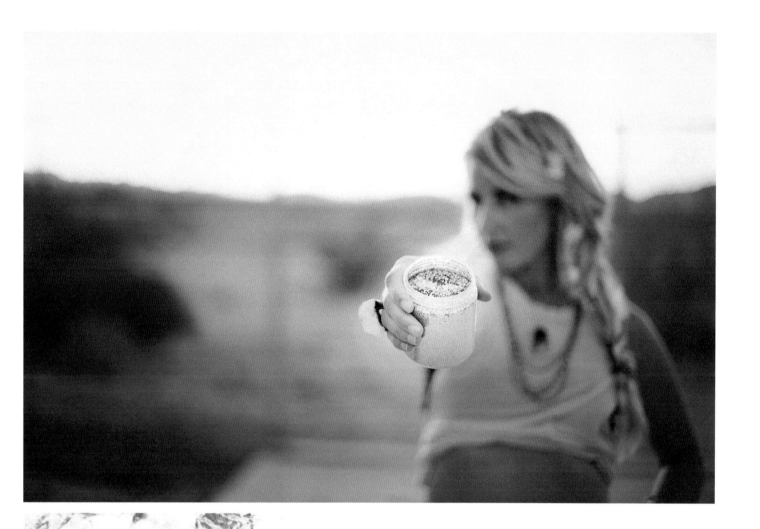

6. So what do I eat to piss this glitter you speak of?

Simple—nourishment with a side of enjoying life. Eat more nutrients; eat fewer ingredients.

Just. Eat. Real. Food.

#jerf. Choose food with the least amount of ingredients and as close to a food's natural state as possible.

Imagine stocking your fridge and pantry only with items your great-great-grandmother could have. Imagine yourself asking your great-great grandmother if she wanted a bite of your Fiber One bar.

Could you just picture how confused she would be about this "food" in a weird wrapper that allegedly is supposed to help her poop? I mean, right?

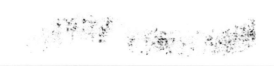

My Staples

- Lots of Clean Meats (protein).
- Good fats.
- Greens.
- Pasture raised or grass-fed butter.
- Full-fat cheese, preferably raw.
- Coconut everything.
- Carbs from veggies and a dash of fruit.
- Red wine and dark chocolate, though I try to stick to weekends for wine so I don't "need it" nightly . . . which I used to . . . champers with the beezies.
- Rinse with LOTS of water.

This is not a diet. This is a way of life. This is about joy in all aspects of your life. This is about nourishment.

This is not a case of calories in and calories out. This is a case of eating foods that best digest, as determined partly due to our genetic makeup, and deliver nutrients to all the cells in our bodies.

This is a case of your body's ability to store fat versus burn fat based on the quality of calories consumed, not just the amount.

I am not asking you to starve yourself; I am encouraging you to eat good proteins and fat, potentially reduce carbs, detox from all forms of sugar, and allow your body to react to insulin as it should.

When we lower our carb intake and teach our body to use fat for fuel, we stop mistaking insulin levels for ravenous hunger and can begin to truly feel what hunger is . . . and eventually see our abs.

There is no magic pill or wrap or shake or tea. There is no calorie counting. There is only listening to the needs of your body.
And every**body** is different.

These are the things I personally eat after years of experimenting with my diet. I cannot tolerate processed carbs or grains, or too many carbs from even fruit. When I eat more carbs, I see more chunk and experience more pain.

My naturally thin husband, however, can just handle more carbs, like a bowl of ice cream with chocolate sauce MULTIPLE nights a week.

At the end of the day, how many calories we consume matters, but what matters much, MUCH more is what that food does IN and TO our bodies.

Some calories fuel. Some calories make us want to consume more energy than we expend. Some calories cause us to store them as fat. Some calories never suffice the needs of our cells, which tricks our body into starvation and storage.

Hopefully, you will learn to devour calories that nourish different needs and provide fuel.

Hear this:

Cutting calories alone will signal cortisol (stress hormone) to HOLD ON to the chub you already have stored. Calorie deficits also signal leptin (hunger hormone) to fire up your hunger in a way that literally makes us HANGRY and very difficult to control. Eat good foods when you are hungry, and you will never torture your soul with calorie counting or binging again.

We want calories that deliver nutrients, burn fat, and give us the energy we need to rock the shit out of our days.

USELESS NOTE:

I hate that hubs eats processed junk like Doritos on the reg, and I am 98.3% certain this hatred is fueled for my desire for him to be as healthy as possible our entire lives together and not due to sheer envy.

Jury is still out.

NERD NOTES:

You do have to burn more than you consume for weight loss, but the quality of DIGESTIVE calories is more important than the amount of just any old calories. Eat calories that your body can digest, move, and goddammit enjoy life.

Without further ado and in order of personal importance, here are the ways I eat for the healthiest version of me. I encourage you to explore my suggestions but ALWAYS listen to your body.

We are not the same. Your needs are different than mine. The general principles I follow will most likely help, but there may be adjustments you will need to make on your road to your best self. With love.

Cook.
Clean.
Do something!

Your kitchen is your medicine cabinet. Your dining room is your therapist.

1. Your kitchen is your medicine cabinet. Your dining room table is your therapist.

Cook your meals.

I believe all of my health problems developed because as a society we have broken up with the kitchen and are constantly on the hunt for "quick fixes." Anything that takes longer than five minutes to prepare is too long, and our bodies and families are paying for it.

I will not even argue the fast food industry has destroyed our waistline, but the microwave. We have created a society where shortcuts are not fast enough, and we simply do not take the time to map the road ahead, nor learn from the road behind us.

You have to slow down. You have to start cracking eggs again, roasting meat for hours, and sitting down to meals together. If you read nothing else in this entire book or anything on nutrition, read this.

My biggest piece of advice is this: Cooking your meals is non-negotiable. It was not until I personally started preparing 90% of all of my meals did I see a change in my body. A variety of factors were at play, but if you ask me, the moment I started tying my apron I started shredding into a better quality bod, which both I and the hubs appreciated.

I do not care what you cook or how you prepare it, just buy fresh ingredients. Start there. Even if you ignore everything else in this book, I know what you will serve yourself; your soul will not be fried in canola oil or injected with high fructose corn syrup. It will hopefully be free of chemicals and thickeners, and for me that is enough for now.

So, Betty, start cooking! If you want to see your abs, they really are made in the kitchen so keep reading. Put love into your meals like your grandmother did. Don't just warm them up.

Funny story. My Grandma Betty was a wonderful cook. She believed in whole foods and taking care of her husband and family through food. She told me that I needed to cook more for my husband so she offered to teach me how.

A few months before she passed we attempted a meatloaf together. She kicked me out of the kitchen after about ten minutes, laughed at me for being hopeless, and finished the meal herself because hubs was coming over to eat; she could not bear the thought of him eating whatever it was that I was trying to create.

This is one of my greatest memories of her. We have a rather crazy family, and I do not mean crazy in the sense that we are all loud and talk over each other. We are that, too. We just are actually crazy and have trouble being in the same room together. But one thing my grandma knew was that we could always find our way together over a good meal.

She made the BEST spaghetti, and when I abandoned processed carbs she still would make me batches from scratch to have on hand to pour over my broccoli. I am no where near the cook that she was, but I would like to believe part of her legacy lives on within me every time I attempt a new recipe for hubs and Wubbas.

It was very important to her that we women found time to cook for our men and children. Call this old fashioned, but I believe it is one of the secrets to my very happy marriage. Hubs is actually more of the chef in our family than I am, but we eat almost all of our dinners at home together.

Sometimes dinner is at 9 p.m. after we are both done with work, but it is the one time we have together every day; that is how we attack life together—one bite at a time. We turn the TV off and the conversation up.

Make real foods available fast.

I cook a couple of nights a week preparing a lot of protein, greens, and sides for the days ahead. That way I can just heat a few things up in the oven or the stove, and we are ready to eat within minutes.

My life is not conducive to cooking for hours each night, so I carve out time every Sunday and about Wednesday to make sure we have things on hand in the days between. I also love me a crockpot meal and have shared my favorite crocks in the recipe section.

I think Grandma Betty would be proud of the cook I am today though she would tell me, "Now if it were me, I would add more salt, and don't be afraid of butter!" You butter believe it, Granny! I love and miss you but am thankful to feel you in my kitchen every day.

Sobremesa:

The time spent after a meal, sitting around and talking to the other people sharing the meal with you.

There is no English equivalent to the Spanish word Sobremesa, and maybe that is part of our problem.

Nourish your gut.

2. Nourish your gut.

To aid the digestion of all the foods you eat and to give your immune system a righteous boost, I suggest getting some probiotics and/or prebiotics into that belly daily! Prebiotics and probiotics both essentially promote good gut bacteria.

You NEED the good bacteria to keep out the bad bacteria, to keep inflammation at bay, and really to keep your immune system strong. Bacteria (most bacteria) are actually really good for our bodies. Believe it or not, we actually have more bacteria in our bodies than human cells.

We live in an anti-bacterial on your keychain world; this almost sounds counterintuitive. We have been told bacteria are the enemy, and disease spreads in an unsanitary environment. While this is true and health codes have come a long way to prevent the spread of disease, we have along the way destroyed much of the bacteria we need in our bodies to function and thrive.

Bacteria is essential for gut and immune health, so whip out that jar of pickles and go to town. BUT, not all pickles are created equally. Most pickles at the grocery store contain high fructose corn syrup or sugar, so avoid these nuggets.

I love "Bubbies" pickles and sauerkraut. "Bubbies" make my tummy very, very happy.

Gut Nourishing Foods for Good Gut Bacteria

- Sauerkraut
- Pickles
- Jicama
- Kimchi
- Kombucha
- Full-fat yogurt
- Kefir
- Onions (bleggh!)
- Garlic

Yummy fermented foods like pickles, kombucha in a wine glass, full fat yogurt (preferably unprocessed or homemade), kefir, and my personal favorite sauerkraut will make the bacteria in your gut happy.

Prebiotics also promote a smokin' haute gut. Foods like jicama, onions, and garlic provide the prebiotic inulin (a type of fiber), which gut flora consume, and help to keep the flora alive and well!

Sometimes when I am feeling hungry after a full meal, one delightful Bubbies pickle crushes my need. I will even dip jicama in my Beezy Sauce (see recipes) for a gut flora loving dessert. It is like my body screams, "Give me some bacteria and enzymes so I can break down all the delights you ate for dinner!" Yep. I, too, realize how odd that sounds, especially reading it out loud.

Gut Supporting Supplements

Fermented Cod Liver Oil
Prebiotic
Gelatin

Supplement your diet to really soothe that gut. Wubbas and I both consume fermented cod liver/butter oil blend and powdered probiotics every day. Fermented cod liver/butter oil is kind of like our multivitamin being a good source of fat-soluble vitamins A, D, E, and K2. It is also rich in EPA and EHA (the stuff they add to every baby formula basically on the market), and is very important for brain and the nervous system.

A prebiotic supplement is something I have found has helped me tremendously with digestion and gut health. Wubbas was also on antibiotics when he was first born, which I quickly decided he did not need, so I am pretty militant on making sure he gets his daily prebiotic to help repopulate all the good gut bacteria developing in his wittle immune and digestive system.

Pssst. Check out the Three-Week Gut Check!

"Fermented cod liver oil is the one supplement I think nearly everyone can benefit from. I've seen it clear acne, lift depression, balance hormones, and reverse autoimmunity. I use it myself and recommend it to all of my patients."

— Dr. Chris Kresser, L.Ac.

Drink water,
all day
erry day.

3. Drink water, all day errry day.

- Water = abs
- Water = hormonal function
- Water = muscle health
- Water = cellular health
- Water = healthy body

Water = delivery of nutrients = properly functioning organs = increased oxygen uptake.

Dehydration = fat storage = lethargy = sickness.

Back to some caveman shit; throughout history draughts happen just before famine. So our bodies adapted to believe that when we are low on water, a famine could be fast approaching. Bring on the fat storage!

Preventing chub rub storage is enough for me to get through a good 10+ glasses of water every day. Just for kicks though, you should know that muscle tissue is composed of nearly 80% water and helps deliver proper nutrients and energy to all of the cells of your body.

Inadequate hydration limits the delivery of oxygen to tissues and can seriously lower blood pressure, which can cause a host of issues. Moreover, hydration is essential for the proper circulation and interaction of hormones, AND your ability to build muscle properly (10.).

Keeping things simple; all systems of your body need water to operate efficiently, and dehydration and fat storage are pretty much BFFs.

Drink. Water. I aim for a good 70 ounces or more a day.

Eat food,
not packaging.

4. Eat food, not packaging.

For the love of God, stop counting calories and start counting nutrients. If it is green, eat it! If man made it, skip it.

Find veggies you like and find a way that you like them cooked. I personally shower in brussel sprouts almost every day (see recipes). But before you run to the cold section at Whole Foods for a green drink, a juice that has agave or 45 grams of sugar in it per serving, does not a fat burning machine make. Sugar, sugar, sugar, masking itself as greens.

Hear this. We can no longer single symptom treat and single supplement dose our bodies. This means we need to approach food as medicine, because it is. It is our nourishment, our survival, and it determines whether we thrive or wither. We know we want to eat blueberries because they give us antioxidants, but this is not enough.

Macronutrients (fat, protein, and carbohydrates) as well as the micronutrients (vitamins, minerals, and other beneficial chemicals) in food work best in combination with each other.

We know we need calcium, so we order some amazing calcium wonder supplement online. But did you know if you are deficient in vitamin D, you will not absorb the calcium pills (and many other nutrients) you have been popping for better bones?

The solution is not to take a vitamin D supplement and a calcium supplement; the solution is to eat a variety of foods with an array of vitamins, minerals, and nutrients. The only way to do this is to eat a variety of vegetables, fruits, tubers (sweet potatoes, etc.), and good, clean meats. And a good source of fat because MANY nutrients are fat soluble, meaning you need fat to actually USE the nutrients!

Food sensitivities, health conditions, and even chronic stress can impact how we assimilate nutrients. If we are not absorbing nutrients, we are starving the cells of our body. If we are starving the cells of our body, we are storing fat and making lots of room for disease. Yum!

Beating a dead horse here, but our bodies need nutrients for all of our cells to function properly and to avoid tricking our bodies into thinking we are starving. So do your damnedest to add greens and colorful veggies to every meal to consume lots of delightful nutrients.

My favorite thing on the whole planet is to wake up, drink my buttered coffee (see recipes), and then take the Wubbas for a walk, a dash of vitamin D, and a delightful green drink from Señor Mangos (See recipes, Spicy Bitch is my fave). Starting my morning with a little fat and greens seems to work wonders.

My advice to you is to GET more nutrients in your food, nutrients from a variety of meats, vegetables, fruits, and tubers. From there, test to see if you have any adverse reactions to dairy, grains, and legumes.

Sure this will take time, but if you are miserable, truly want to shed some fat, and feel better in your body, this is a worthy road to travel.

A few idears (ay-deer-s-uh) to enjoy more greens:

- Cook greens in butter, ghee, left over bacon grease or coconut oil.
- Store your leftover bacon grease in a glass or ceramic container—rumor says it stays good forever on the counter when covered, but I recommend placing it in the fridge.
- Bacon fat could be used to make eggs, sauté veggies, or rub on a roasted chicken.
- Make your greens taste delightful.
- Cook greens and add bacon, sausage, or insert favorite animal fat here.
- Get creative; add nuts, animal fats, and fruit to green sides.
- Add a handful of spinach or mixed greens to a smoothie.
- Chop up a bunch of veggies every Sunday to have on hand and then add them to any salad, casserole, or egg dishes you make.

Nerd Alert:

For more on some the most important vitamins and nutrients you could be missing and how to actually get AND absorb them, check out the Weston A. Price Foundation.

NERD NOTES:

- Eat more nutrients = less fat storage
- Counting calories + not eating real food = intense cravings + chub rub

Limit carbs and/or determine which ones you digest best.

5. Limit carbs and/or determine how and which ones you digest best.

I am not sure if you have heard me so far, but our modern diet is drowning in sugar—glucose broken down from carbs, unable to be stored and magically transformed into chub rub.

We believe that we need to eat less to weigh less, but instead we are just depriving our cells of nutrients, thus teaching our bodies to store more fat. I have learned to live a life empty of "whole grains" but full of love and the abs I once knew. My favorite form of carbs comes in veggies (insert eye roll here).

No one actually loves getting their carbs entirely from veggies (and some fruits), but I do really love sweet potatoes, yams, and butternut squash. Of which I will have close to two servings a day, but it is always the last thing I add to my plate after the greens, protein, and fat (See recipes for sweet delights.).

Now and then, I will add some quinoa and wild rice to a dish if I am dining with others, but it really is a now and then delight, and I recommend it when you are in a more active mode of your life.

My husband says that I "demonize" carbs, and maybe I do; but like I said, this is what works for ME. These are MY beliefs based off of personal trial and error and devouring words on words on words and studies on studies on studies about the role of nutrition on our health.

That said, I do believe some people can get away with eating more carbs than others. I do believe some people cannot. I know that every person has to figure that out for themselves, and they will not find the answer in any book.

I think I "demonize" carbs and whole-ish grains because I'm angry having been misled my whole life regarding their importance and role in my life. Excess glucose in my body (broken down from simple and complex carbs) always leaves my body a little chunky and a lot achy. The arthritis I am certain I got rid of reminds me that inflammation is easy to flare up again with too much sugar.

The thing is, a carb is a carb is a carb, and in your body, glucose is glucose is glucose.

Grains, fructose (sugar found in fruit or honey), lactose (sugar found in dairy), or a mix of fructose and dextrose (found in plain table sugar) all circulate as glucose in your body once you metabolize it.

If there is any extra glucose floating around in the body that we are not immediately using to replenish glycogen stores, it is stored as fat.

I love fruit. It is delightful and nutritious. I just cannot have a ton of it. I aim for one to three servings a day if I need the extra energy. When the mood is right, I will do fruit for my nightcap sweet tooth, but I usually like a little fruit in the morning after my coffee or with a lunch salad or as a pick-me-up with a handful of nuts or nut butter.

Enjoy it, and just remember it does break down to sugar in your body. If you are choosing between fruit and some processed sugary crap, however, I promise your body will better know how to use the energy from fruit than the crap.

Learn to listen to your body.

Fact. Sometimes we "crave" fruit because we are dehydrated, and the blend of sugar and the water content in fruit makes us feel better momentarily. Learn your hunger signals = meet your abs.
Some people say to me, "Well aren't you just doing the Atkins diet?"

No. Sure, Dr. Atkins advocated a high fat, low-carb diet based on tremendous science. But Atkins fell short in two ways. Number one is the quality of foods allowed on the diet plan, or lack there of. And two is lifetime sustainability.

Thinking logically, any type of fat without the presence of carbs will allow your body to start burning fat instead of sugar (glycogen) and help you lose weight quickly. HOWEVER, when your fat sources are cheddar sticks, overly processed and junky beef jerky, and roasted canola oil-drenched cashews, your body will eventually feel starved for nutrients and have difficulty digesting, which will cause intense cravings and the abrupt end of the diet.

Most people lose a lot of weight quickly on Atkins, but when they realize it's not sustainable over a lifetime, defeat packs the pounds back on much faster than they lost them. They never actually teach themselves how to eat, how to thrive and feel ridiculous in their own skin. They just feel thinner, and for a while that is enough.

Hear this: I do not believe it is good for your body or hormones to be extremely low carb all the time.

I actually learned this the only way I know how to learn, the hard way. I was extremely low carb for almost an entire year, sure with indulgences here and there but for the most part carbless, avoiding fruit and anything that would "spike my insulin."

And it took a serious toll on my hormones AND my mental health, quite frankly.

What I learned was that my body does need carbs, just not a ton of carbs. Fruit makes my skin much happier, and not restricting an entire food group liberates my soul.

If you are looking to lose weight quickly, dropping the carbs will help. But after a few weeks, you need to eat some carbs and reset your leptin levels so your body does not think you are starving. Here's a great read on carb refers with juicy facts.

After that, it is all about moderation and listening to your body. Eat a good amount of protein. There is a reason why bodybuilders and figure competitors eat a ton of protein, it helps build and maintain muscles, and helps you feel fuller, longer.

Add some delightful veggies and fruit to your plate.

Eat some good fats, and eat a good source of carbs, all of which in moderation. Do not exclude or overeat any single macronutrient (protein, carbs, fat).

Nerd Sugar

Fact. Your body cannot store that much glycogen, but it can store a ton of fat. Our bodies evolved using fat for energy. Our ability to store glycogen (sugar from carbs) is actually very limited, but our ability to store fat for survival due to times where food was scarce and we did not eat every two to three hours to "stabilize our blood sugar" is endless.

So what does that mean? You can tell your modern day nutritionist that if we evolved relying on carbs for energy and no fat, we would have died because we could not store food to survive winters, war, and famine. Your body wants energy from GOOD fats and proteins, not sugar.

Fact. Something beyond the actual number of calories is playing a role in how the body uses energy and burns fat. Studies even show that those who consume a very low carbohydrate diet actually end up burning more energy and thus fat in the long run (11.).

You've heard of nutrients. You've heard of calories in, calories out. But have you heard the *alternative hypothesis*? That something greater is going on than simply calories. In fact, nutrients, anti-nutrients, hormones, irritants, and the list goes on and on, are all at play here.
And they all can affect your ability to burn or store calories.

Alternative hypothesis -

Obesity is a growth disorder, just like any other growth disorder, and fat accumulation is determined not by the balance of calories consumed and expended but by the effect of specific nutrients on the hormonal regulation of fat metabolism (12.).

Therefore, your goal is to assess how your body digests and uses its calories for energy. Are you eating too many or too few calories? Are you eating calories that you are digesting? Your genetic makeup and lifestyle may allow you to shower in tons of fruit, oats, and even plain old white sugar. To which I say, you is a lucky bitch!

Like one of my bestest little beezies Tara; she is a conundrum. She is almost five feet tall. Rides motorcycles. Runs six miles a day. And CANNOT live without toast. Her abs? To die for. I love to hate her.

For the majority of us beezies, however, I am willing to wager that limiting your carb intake will help your overall health and ab lines in the long run.

For those of you crazy calorie counters and carb measurers, which I personally think is a waste of time and will drive you nuts, I would aim to reduce your daily carb intake to about 50-100 grams if you don't get off your donk much, and 100-150 grams if you are highly active.

Basically, you want to reduce your carb intake relative to your body's demands. This takes practice, but will most definitely assist in fat loss and greater health. A good rule of thumb is if your weight is staying the same or steadily decreasing (if and only if it needs to) your carb level is close to on point.

A Note on Keto

If you want to put your body into Nutritional Ketosis, you need to be eating less than 50 grams a day. I find that my magic keto number is really about 30 or less grams of carbs a day. 30 grams of carbs is about how many carbs you would consume in ONE banana. Just sayin'.

Oh, and ketosis is basically a metabolic state that causes ketones to be produced by the liver to provide energy to the body, as a result of shifting from burning sugar to burning fat. In contrast, a state of glycolysis is where glycogen (sugar) provides energy to the body.

You have to have very, **very** minimal amounts of carbs (glycogen stores) in order to allow your body to get into a state of ketosis. If done correctly, your body can really burn through a lot of fat, without hampering your energy. In fact, when I am in a state of Nutritional Ketosis, my energy is magnetic!

However, I do have one word of caution when it comes to putting your body into ketosis. Although it can be very effective for quick fat loss, it is NOT something you should do all the time. Overtime your hormones and adrenals will rebel against you if you abuse this method of weight loss.

You do need carbs in your life. You need to be careful not to make any certain food the enemy of all time.

In a Nutshell

In reducing carbs and eliminating toxins in your body from processed garbage, you will learn what and how much of it your body needs to eat. There is no greater feeling in the world than fueling your body with nutrients dipped in bacon grease. True story morning glory, cook greens in left over bacon grease. #nomnomnom

Bonus:

For a scientific dissertation on Nutritional Ketosis, I again direct you to Peter Attia's Eating Academy.

NERD NOTES:

- Any carb you put in your mouth = glucose in your body
- Too much glucose in your body = fat + disease
- Less glucose in your bloodstream = abs + hormonal balance
- Starving yourself of carbs for a lifetime = hormonal ruckus

Eat good, clean meats, fish and eggs!

6. Eat good, clean meats, fish, and eggs!

My former vegetarian self would baulk at this, but it is my belief that you need meat.

You do. Really. But you need good meat from healthy animals. My hormones, fat stores, and happiness really came about when I broke up with soy and started going steady with grass-fed beef.

There is no greater love than when hubs makes me a grass-fed burger patty, lettuce wrapped with a side of baked sweet potato fries. No greater joy. No greater love. No greater burger. He makes the goddam best burgers. Mouth watering. Should be writing not salivating.
Sorry, okay back to the meats!

Fill your plate with good clean meats and fish. Think grass-fed/pasture raised red meats, organic free-range chicken or turkey, and fish that is NOT pond raised or farmed (check the label) as much as humanly possible. I am a meat snob and won't touch it if it is not organic and/or grass-fed.

Why organic, free range, green-fed, grass-fed or pasture raised? What's wrong with farm-raised fish? Simple. Nutrients. Toxins. Digestibility.

Back to our science lesson. Nutrients are essential for your body to digest food, fuel your immune, hormonal and energy systems, and to allow your body to send the correct signals for what it needs.

Antibiotics and tons of other junk modern farming has blessed us with really do not sit well in your body. Antibiotics, chemicals, and toxins found in your cheap meat interfere with hormones and enzymatic activity in your bod, costing you a chain of dangerous health reactions over time.

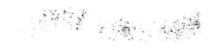

USELESS NOTE:

My hubs likes to fight me on this one; go ahead and watch the documentary "Frankensteer" if you would like to be persuaded.

When animals live as they were intended, grazing the good earth, they are the healthiest forms of themselves and naturally consume the nutrients their bodies need. Just like when we were doing more caveman shit, walking everywhere and eating what the land had to offer us, our bodies were healthier.

When animals are shoved into an itty bitty space with hundreds of others and fed the most cost effective, fattening, antibiotic drowned chow possible, the meat that ends up in your Big Mac is not the way nature intended.

It actually becomes very difficult to digest and causes a host of issues in your own body, beyond the assault on your hips.

Bonus: When an animal is raised in an environment where they can graze the good land, they actually consume a ton of nutrients that YOU need and can obtain from their meat. Yes, you still need vegetables, but you can get a TON of nutrients and protein and good fats from HEALTHY animals.

Think of the big beef industry. It is a massive, big business beast. It is efficient and cost effective. They really do not give a shit about your health or safety; they care about fattening up their product, keeping it alive long enough to get it to your plate, and turning a profit.

The conditions animals live in are so terrible; they are injecting them with tons of antibiotics just because farmers are able to do so. "Umm yeah, can I get a number two, animal style with an extra side of antibiotics and a compromised immune system please? Hold the cheese!"

Note: I really hate fear-based nutrition books, blogs and forums, but . . . if I can instill one piece of fear in you, it is to routinely consume meat from giant suppliers. Again, I direct you to "Frankensteer" if you would like to learn more.

Here is my advice with meat: avoid conventionally raised meats. Honestly, a vegetarian diet is better than eating crappy meat at least for your digestion and immune system. Though I believe you will be missing nutrients and not living up to optimal hormonal function, just like I was in my cranky kale-noshing-tofu-loving stupor.

Honor the whole animal.

Now while you may not want to think about where things come from for whatever reason, I do believe if you eat meat, you eat meat and you should consider honoring the whole animal. The animal has already given its life for your nourishment so why scoff at the other less glamorous parts of consumption? They have amazing healing properties, and I am thankful for their sacrifice.

Hippy primal shit, I know.

Fact. Bone broth is an AMAZING source of gelatin. Gelatin is largely composed of the amino acids glycine and proline, which many people do not consume in adequate amounts as they are found in the bones, fibrous tissues and organs of animals and as a population, we do not consume these parts as much anymore. These amino acids are needed not only for proper skin, hair and nail growth, but for optimal immune function and weight regulation.

Ever wonder why chicken soup was the staple for healing after a cold or a flu? Because traditionally it was made from boiling down the bones and feet of the animal, which made it rich with gelatin and helped those who were ill bounce back quickly. Chicken soup in a can, is not the same though its warmth maybe comforting.

All right, getting off my high horse, but I urge you to explore different cuts of meat and look into making your own bone broth. Double dare you.

If you are not ready for that type of gnarly in your kitchen, I would recommend looking into a gelatin supplement to make delightful desserts and add to your gut and immune health (See resources for recommended brands.).

Eats the Meats and What to Buy:

Beef
Organic + grass-fed or green-fed ONLY. Cows that are fed a traditional diet of grains and antibiotics end up becoming a very, very difficult fat to digest. Grass-fed and green-fed cows supply a much more digestible and nutritious source of protein, good fats, antioxidants, vitamins, and minerals. If you do not have access to grass-fed or green-fed beef, I would stick to organic poultry and wild caught fish and skip the beef.

Poultry
Organic pasture raised is best. Organic free range is next. Organic is third in line. After that, I would skip it.

Fish
Wild caught, not farm raised. It has been said that farm-raised fish contain more toxins than many conventional raised meats.

Eggs
Preferably pasture raised which makes them rich in antioxidants, good fats, vitamins, and—for the calories—a lot of protein. Pastured eggs are typically double in the protein content because they eat bugs, greens, and the wonderful things nature intended. Pasture raised eggs are best. Organic free-range come next. Commercial eggs are shit, and I suggest avoiding them.

Bones
Use the bones of animals or the leftovers from your roasted poultry to make bone broth! It is amazingly high in gelatin, which is SO good for your joints, immune, and digestive systems.

NERD NOTES:

- Healthy animals = healthy humans
- Unhealthy animals = unhealthy humans

Eat fat.
Drink raw milk.
Maybe avoid grains.

7. Eat fat. Drink raw milk. Maybe avoid grains.

Before you hate me, let me just again reiterate that some people digest grains just fine. Some people have no problem with dairy. Some people eat a bag of nuts a day and look amazing. All of these things are huge big fat no-no's in the paleo world. But we ain't crawling in their cave so it's just fine.

You should, however, think about their reasoning and, perhaps, use it as a base for your new way of life. Personally, when I stripped out grains, dairy, nuts, and legumes and focused on meat, veggies, fruit, and tubers (like sweet potatoes, braugh), I became much healthier. Then I experimented with raw dairy and did great for a while; but when my diet gets way out of control and I am too cocky with anything I goddam feel like eating, dairy gives me allergies alongside the other crap in my body.

So hot shit, this chapter is to give you some tools and thoughts about discovering how you react to grains, legumes, nuts, and dairy. Fat is non-negotiable. Eat it. Mmmm, butter.

Low-fat Wet Dreams

So I know you probably have heard two things over and over in the last fifteen years or so. Eat your whole grains and avoid fat.

REVERSE this in your mind forever. The low-fat trend was really just Frito-Lay's marketing wet dream that lets you feel good about crushing bags of "baked" low-fat potato chips. You may be eating entirely low-fat, but you will indeed still be fat, missing nutrients and craving more low-fat crap.

Grains that are not traditionally prepared, via soaking and fermenting, have been shown to cause nutrient deficiencies, mess with digestion, contribute to autoimmune diseases, and contain opioids which literally make them addicting (13.). Research has even shown that the longer an animal is fed grains, the more nutrients are lost (14.).

Remember our science lesson? Less nutrients = fat storage. Toxins = fat storage. This is why I avoid MOSTLY all grains, unless they are in my mom's famous coconut oatmeal chewy cookies; then I am showering in that shit.

Studies have shown that removing grains, processed dairy, and legumes (more carbs and difficult to digest) while increasing protein helps your body stabilize insulin (15.). We want insulin to be able to do its job supplying energy and nutrients, so avoiding foods that cause it to rise to the occasion and start racketeering with our fat storage is the key.

And our good friend fat is actually good for you. Many major studies have proven that the low-fat diet Bible has been telling us lies, and the diet simply does not work. The low-fat diet has been put to the test in several huge randomized controlled trials. It does not cause any weight loss over a period of seven and a half years, and it has literally no effect on heart disease or cancer (16.).

The Chubby Anti-Nutrient Story of Whole Grains, Legumes, and Nuts

Whole grains are not meant to be digested in their original state. Nature wants them to stay in tact so animals can graze them and poop them out somewhere else, populating their seed across the land. Whole grains thus contain chemicals that inhibit your ability to absorb nutrients, and wreak havoc on your gut when they are consumed in excess and not digested properly.

For example, whole grains can inhibit your body's ability to absorb and utilize vitamin D, calcium, zinc, and iron (17.). So even if you are getting a reasonable amount of sun and eating an otherwise nutritious diet, whole grains can literally block your ability to digest and use those nutrients for energy and cell function.

Chuuu telling me all that kale I choked down was all for not?

Maybe, baby.

Here is what the caveman paleo folk say: You should not eat grains or legumes or nuts because they carry anti-nutrients, basically compounds that prevent you from breaking them down so that the plant can be pooped out and grow again. Yep.

I am totally not even a little bit interested in debating that issue. Personally, I do not eat a lot grains, because I really do not think my body digests them well, and they tend to carry a heavy load of glucose in my blood stream, which is not great for me, my abs, my skin, or my happiness. Now and then I will have a little oatmeal, which I have SOAKED overnight and I seem to survive. SO that is cool. Just not every day.

Point is, PLANTS contain anti-nutrients. Not just the plants the paleo community decided would. That is how a plant survives and propagates, but this does not mean, however, that you should ALWAYS avoid grains, legumes, and nuts.

Too much of something is almost always toxic. For example, we can all go ahead and agree spinach is a healthy food. Spinach does carry a small amount of oxalates, which is an anti-nutrient. If you eat a ton of spinach, eventually the oxalates will start to irritate your gut, at which time you should listen to your body and back off. But should I stop eating spinach ENTIRELY because of this?

No. Spinach is a wonderful nutrient.

Kale contains typically more phytic acid than nuts, which the paleo primal world will tell you to run from.

Dark leafy greens are good for you, right? They just do not taste good enough to be bad for you!

Yeah, mostly, they are good for you. But some people with thyroid issues cannot tolerate dark leafy greens, and it can actually make their condition worse. This is also the case for a variety of nutrients. If spinach is the only lettuce you eat three times a day, seven days a week, your body might get sick of it and stop breaking it down.

Fiber at one point was considered an anti-nutrient, and humans were urged to avoid it. But now we know, dietary fiber is actually very good for you and helps you DIGEST your food.

Conclusion:

Soak your nuts and grains.

I guess my point is, you have to decide for yourself how your body digests certain foods. I would make the case for soaking, sprouting, and heating grains, beans, and nuts is a safe bet as it does reduce the contents of anti-nutrients. But I am not convinced the science to date can tell you that you should 100% avoid it entirely, for a lifetime!

The Skinny on Fat

Fat literally helps you burn, baby, burn. Eating a moderate/digestible fat, moderate protein, and moderate to low-carb diet teaches your body to burn fat instead of sugar and is arguably a more efficient use of energy.

Fat burns slow and evenly, so you are fuller longer and just feel better throughout the day. Carbs burn quickly and are gone quickly, leaving you feeling empty and reaching for more and never getting the nutrients or energy you truly crave.

When I drink coffee (every day), I sometimes blend it with butter (ghee or grass-fed), sea salt, and coconut oil, or I add full fat, pasture raised, organic heavy whipping cream and cinnamon. YUMM-O in my TUMM-O. The mix of fat and caffeine has a more systemic effect on my body, and I have energy for longer, as the caffeine does not rush in and out of me like a regular cup (See recipes for buttery delights).

Keep in mind however, if you are throwing butter and coconut oil in your coffee everyday, and having fat and a ton of carbs at every other meal, this does not a fat loss recipe make. Like I said earlier, too much of any one macronutrient (protein, fat, carbs) is not a good idea.

Burn Fat

It is difficult to explain if you have never switched your body from burning sugar to fat. But you actually start to understand your hunger signals and most primal needs. I know when my body needs more water, when it needs greens or fruit because it is missing nutrients, or when it needs some good bacteria from foods like pickles to aid digestion. When your body only burns sugar, your body craves sugar and it masks true needs like hydration.

So, Fatty McFat-Phat, make sure you are eating high quality fats and avoid vegetable oils like the plague. It's crap; accept it. Vegetable oils make you want to believe they are healthy because they have "vegetables" in their name—just like fat makes you want to think it is terrible for you because it has the unfortunate name of fat.

However, good saturated fat like coconut oil and grass-fed butter will not cause your arteries to harden or pack on the pounds; they actually help your brain function and help you look mo bettah naked by teaching your body to BURN fat (18.). They will also help fill you up faster and prevent you from gorging in the calorie fest.

Vegetable oils, on the other hand, are likely genetically modified, making them extremely difficult for your body to digest; and when they coat otherwise nutritious foods like nuts, they irritate your gut and add inches to your donk! There are two things I cannot live without: anything coconut and eggs (Bahhh! Oh and coffee, so three things.). My husband believes that I single handedly keep the coconut industry in business, we have chickens in our backyard, and I have three different vessels that brew coffee in different ways (if you care).

Coconuts provide good fat, have tremendous holistic properties, help curb sweet cravings, and rumor has it the oil is a delightful substitute for some sort of jelly you don't spread on toast, whose name I believe starts with KY. Think about it. Ahhhh! There it is.

I also love me some avocado, fatty fish, and when I have a sweet tooth, I will literally eat coconut butter from the jar. No carbs. Yummy texture and oh so satisfying.

Crack Some Eggs

But eggs will raise your cholesterol! Nope, not even a little. Studies show that egg consumption is not associated with heart disease. Whole eggs are amongst the most nutritious foods on the planet, and they actually elevate your good cholesterol (HDL).

When you cook eggs in coconut oil, heaven actually cracks the gate for crazies like you and I just for a brief moment so we can get a whiff of what it might smell like inside.

Fact. Eggs are the perfect food for pregos, nursing mothers, and tots. Eggs are an extremely healthy and economical food, providing complete protein in the whites and a variety of healthy fats in the yolks.

Egg yolks contain large amounts of important nutrients for the brain. A lot of the time, adults and babies are allergic to egg whites but not the yolks, so keep that in mind when feeding your youngins!

Cooking Fats

I like to cook with grass-fed/pasture raised BUTTER, ghee, coconut oil, or avocado oil, and I try to never heat olive oil because it changes the molecular structure and makes it difficult for your body to digest the otherwise wholesome oil.

Go Nuts

I love nuts (That's what she said.), which is not terrible; but after years of being a vegetarian and never actually feeling full, I can drown a bag of cashews in two days for quick energy and satiety. I still buy nuts, but always check the label. If they have vegetable oil or sugar or anything you cannot pronounce, skip it.

If there is any havoc you would like to wreak on your digestion, it's a bag of cashews dipped in canola oil and sugar. Your body will not know how to break them down.

Further, nuts can contain similar anti-nutrients and chemicals that grains house, which make them very difficult to digest. For some people, they are impossible to digest. So it is a good idea to roast your nuts, or even better, soak 'em!

Nuts are covered in phytates. Phytates are an indigestible plant compound that inhibits our enzymes from digesting nuts fully. It is believed that by soaking the nuts in purified water overnight, you'll wash away phytates and make the nuts easily digestible, including the key nutrients you need to boost your energy.

I have soaked nuts, and I have eaten them straight from the bag. I can feel in my bones that my body prefers the former, but sometimes when I am at Trader Joe's, that bag of cashews just ain't gonna survive the car ride home untouched. And I don't die.

Do not depend on nuts (That's not what she said.); have them for a reserve, add them to salads and green sides, but don't depend on them for your nutrients and calories for the day. If you find you are not losing weight or changing much, slowly step away from the nuts, ma'am, and feed your body good meats, greens, and always include a healthy fat.

Just a Little Tip:

The first time I tried avoiding carbs, I did not eat nearly enough fat and wanted to throw myself on the floor, kick, scream, and devour a bag of dark chocolate chips. Nowadays, I have fat with every meal, and I have never felt healthier or FULLER. My hubs gives me the stink eye now for the amount of olive oil I will dress my salad with at times, but my thighs don't seem to mind one bit, and he don't seem to mind my thighs.

Sardinians are nuts.

Fact. Some of the longest living and healthiest humans in the world live on a beautiful island off of Italy, Sardinia, where they love to soak walnuts and drink a ton of raw goat's milk. They also are bronze, beautiful, and get plenty of vitamin D from the sun.

Fact. Men on this island will encourage you to drink Mirto (mee-ur-tooohh), which causes a lot of ruckus and dancing in the moonlight.

Say moo.

Raw Milk

I love milk. Oh my God, do I love milk. A cup of wholesome raw milk after a workout is the greatest reward and gets me through some serious sprints and dreadful burpees now and then.

Ex-squeeze me, did you just say raw milk? Why yes, yes I did. Raw milk promotes the production of a wonderful little compound called "glutathione." The tiny little compound is the Master Antioxidant and Detoxifier of cells, meaning it cleans house, removes toxins, helps burn fat, and breaks down difficult to break down shit. Raw milk also contains probiotics.

Basically, raw milk is really good for your immune and digestive systems. My choice of milk is organic, raw, and pasture raised, and I try to avoid pasteurized milk.

The pasteurization process also reduces the nutritional quality of milk products. Research has shown a decrease in manganese, copper, and iron after heat treatment (19.).

While pasteurized milk does retain some level of nutritional value, it seems that unpasteurized milk is superior in vitamin and mineral content overall. I know, I know, I know you've heard for years that raw milk will make you sick. But really, any food item that is mishandled can make you sick. Raw milk just got a bad name from the way it became so mass-produced so quickly that safety fell by the wayside.

Many people experience digestive and other problems when they consume pasteurized milk, but have no trouble with raw milk. Many researchers believe this is because pasteurizing the milk destroys enzymes and probiotics in the milk that make it digestible.

Consuming raw milk is a decision you have to make on your own, though I urge you to give it a try and find a local farm that supplies raw fresh milk.

Not everyone does well with milk. Some people do better with goat than cow too. So investigate for yourself, my friend.

Cheese

Did I mention cheese? How much do you love cheese? Delightful is the word you are looking for. Cheese contains a lot of the delightful nutrients as milk. Cheese, especially when made from the milk of grass-pastured animals, is a wonderful source of several important nutrients including vitamins A, D, B2, B12, and K2; minerals including calcium, zinc, and phosphorus; and is, of course, a great supply of protein and good-for-you fat!

Not all cheese is created equal, of course. Raw pasture raised is best, organic, and minimally pasteurized is next.

Yogurt

Yogurt. So good for you, full of probiotics and all of the lovely nutrients found in raw milk. Since yogurt is basically milk that has been fermented with time, good bacteria is formed that is amazing for your gut and immune system.

Here's the thing though, we are only talking about FULL-FAT, minimally processed milk. Yoplait is terrible for you. Yoplait and Activia are basically sugar and chemicals dressed in yogurt drag. Throw it away. Buy full-fat organic yogurt. Add some berries and a dash of raw honey. Ohhhh man, you are in for a treat.

When my body is more sensitive to milk, it actually still does great with yogurt thanks to the fermentation and digestibility. Just a tip. Just a tip to see how it feels. Just for a minute.

Whey Protein

Bodybuilders have been buying whey milk literally in the pounds for years as it is an amazing source of protein and allegedly helps you build and repair muscle tissue faster. Even if you do not have access to raw milk and/or you just cannot bring yourself to drink it, you can use a high-quality whey protein that comes from grass-fed cows to receive many of the health benefits!

The protein found in milk is whey protein. Whey is the liquid that separates from the curd during the production of cheese. When the liquid dries into powdered whey, the nutrients become concentrated, and it can be packaged and used in that form.

Whey protein can help you fight off colds and flu because it contains beta-glucans and immunoglobulins, which protect your immune system and support your body's natural detoxification processes.

NOW again, your source of whey protein matters. Try an organic and grass-fed whey that is minimally processed. I have included a few of my faves under "resources." I also have some righteous whey protein shake recipes for you to drool over.

NERD NOTES:

- Fat = good for you
- Grains = bad for your gut = bad for you = SOAK THEM
- Fat + grains = really mess up your digestion
- Fat + veggies + healthy animals = abs
- Raw milk = potentially a super nutrient in your life, but you have to sort out how you digest it

Ditch anything
made
in a lab
or served
in a colorful box.

8. Ditch anything made in a lab or served in a colorful box.

Hopefully, so far, you have learned that we need our food to provide nutrients and for our bodies to be able to use our food for energy. And this means no processed anything. If it comes from a box, it is gone, it is garbage and your metabolism probably has no idea what to do with it. Unless you want those Cheddar Bunnies on your Cheddary Thighs, skip 'em.

Learn this now.

Organic does not translate to "good for you".

Organic simply means you will not find any added toxic shit or pesticides. That said, organic mac and cheese may be toxic to you in the sense that it is a huge amount of carbs married with a huge amount of fat that almost always ends in divorce. Good in your mouth, bad in your belly.

Cut soy out of your life immediately. Soy is particularly one of the highest genetically modified food items in the American diet. It shows up basically like pure mucus in your body and contains a lot of estrogen.

So unless you would like an extra dose of hormones (dangerous if you are at risk for breast cancer), and mucus-y goodness your body will not know how to digest and will probably store it somewhere fun like your belly, skip soy.

Almond milk is a better option, but check the ingredients. You do not want added sugars or thickeners or words you cannot pronounce. Raw milk is best.

One thing that kills me is that to this day, you will always find cans of diet coke at my parent's house. To them, it is just now and then. "It's not like we do drugs or smoke," they tell me. It is the one vice I have truly failed them on.

Diet soda is made of chemicals, chemicals that make you feel good and addicted, but without calories so it is good for you! Just because our mode of measuring is calories and diet soda has no caloric effect on your body, we believe it is a safe diet option. But we are NOT measuring its other effects, and those effects are really only measured with time.

:: Update ::

Since reading and editing a few drafts of this book, I have shamed or at least scurred my folks into removing diet soda from their house. WIN!

Eat. More. Nutrients.

You should be concerned when something has no calories, meaning it provides no energy to your body, no nutrients to your cells. And that means some scientist had to find a way for it not to show up in the test we use to measure foods. It is like having to pee in a cup for your druggie brother. He is still going to smoke weed on parole, and getting away with it will just make him crave it more and more.

Artificial sugars are artificial in your body. Your body does not know how to break them down, so your liver suffers. As you may remember, you need your liver to help you burn energy and to keep your immune system strong. Not to mention when your body does not know what to do with something you ate, guess where it stores it? In your chub. Do not poison that bod of yours.

Now and again, I will add a touch of high quality pure maple syrup (straight from trees in New Hampshire if we are getting scientific), raw honey, Xylitol, granulated Stevia, or coconut sugar to sweeten the deal, and these are all plant-based sweeteners. I do believe raw honey is likely the best option for a touch of sweet. Raw honey actually has a host of healing properties, and in moderation is a good option.

True story, I get canker sores now and again mostly stress induced, a dab of raw manuka honey clears it up quicker and soothes the pain. Placebo? Perhaps, but it works for me, and the proof is in the pudding, honey bear.

NERD NOTES:

- Processed + "Skinny marketing" foods = Chubby for a lifetime
- Nutrients + Not overeating = Healthy AND happy for a lifetime

Indulge.
Skinny dip
in Champagne
and
Fresh Ginger
Juice.

9. Indulge. Skinny Dip in Champagne and Fresh Ginger Juice

Yes, you have to cheat.

You have to enjoy life's culinary wonders like Confetti Cupcake Pop-Tarts, or Sunday night dinners from Roberto's occasionally.

On my path of finding balance in my diet, I had some pretty righteous cheat days filled with Pop-Tarts, champagne, and quesadillas to the point where I was sick and most definitely sabotaged much of the clean eating that took place during the week. I felt guilty with every bite and ill at the end of the day.

Now I indulge in Sunday brunch with the hubs, eating whatever he cooks without complaint. YES, I realize I am stupidly lucky to be married to a man who loves to cook, and I fight him constantly on ingredients. But one meal a week, sometimes two, sometimes three, I shut up, I eat, I love, I enjoy, and it is enough.

Sometimes I need champagne. Sometimes that champagne has fresh juiced ginger in it, which serves no healthy purpose other than the fact that it makes my heart warm and makes cheap champagne drinkable.

I have found if I designate one day to cheat, I overindulge and feel guilty. Now I know most of the time my body needs good, clean food, and a little bit of the time my soul needs to go ahead and skinny dip with quesadillas and my mom's famous chocolate chip cookies in a giant vat of champagne (Mumm Brut if we are getting scientific.).

And I do not feel bad about it. That is the key. Enjoy it, walk away, next meal is green. I do not gain any weight from my "cheats," and I actually believe my body resets itself and craves goodness in my next bite.

Live a little, or you will drown in your quest for perfection. Cry and then drown.

Fact. If you worry about every bite, not only will you drive yourself insane, you will slowly isolate yourself from the rest of the world.

When you are at home, cook your meals and control the ingredients you and your family consume. When you are out and about, enjoy life. You know what the better choices are, so choose them.

Be Smart With Your Cheats

Before you go apeshit with cheat meals, justifying to the world that you are practicing 80/20, set realistic expectations for what a cheat is.

80 percent of the time you are a saint, 20 percent of the time you are making it rain with sugar. I do believe 80/20 is a good ratio to strive for; however, most people tend to overestimate the good side and underestimate the bad, making their ratio really more like 70/30 or even 60/40.

Be real with yourself. As your "health coach," I care what you eat, but lying to me or hiding it only adds chub to your rub, not mine.

Fact. Happiness is good food, a glass of deep red wine a night, and laughter.

*Absent a life of joy, is not a life at all.
Live to nourish all parts of you.*

USELESS NOTE:

I once worked with a man who would "mentally cleanse" himself with shrooms every month or so. He probably really believed he pissed glitter at one time or another.)

NERD NOTES:

- Clean Meat + Good Fats + Greens + Limited Fruit
- Occasional Carbs for Energy + Gut Bacteria + Wine
- Occasionally = Honky Tonk Badonkadonk

7.
WHAT ABOUT A MEAL PLAN?

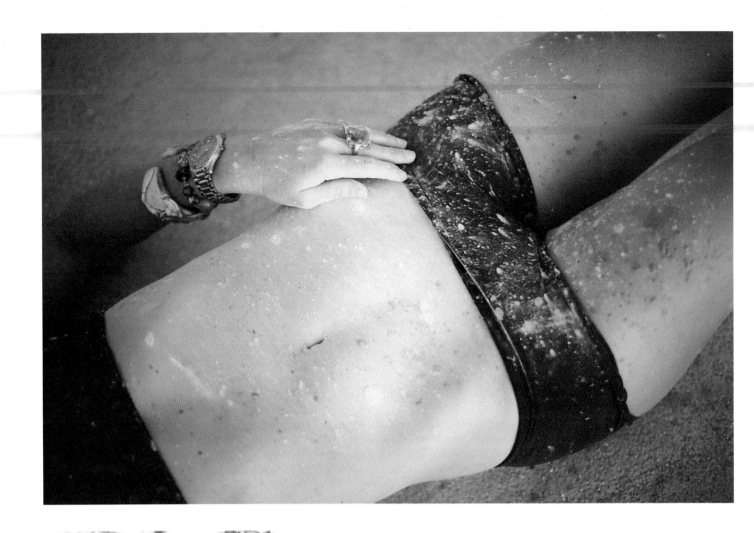

7. What about a meal plan?

In the next chapter, I give you a list of foods to follow and a list of foods to ditch in order to clean up your gut, bloodstream, and hopefully heal your body of inflammation.

This gut check, for me, is actually a way of life, I would say, at least 80 percent of the time. Sure, I indulge now and then, but for the most part, my eats are on point. I have to be, or my PCOS flares up, and I am a miserable chunky, teenage acne ridden beezy.

But as you come out of the gut check, the amount of each given thing you should and should not eat has to come from your own intuitions. As a former serial dieter and cardio addict, this statement would piss off my former self.

I do not expect you to eat like you are in the gut check phase the rest of your life, but I hope you come back to it when you know your body needs it. The gut check will help you feel what your body needs overtime.

My plan for you is as follows:

- Start with the three-week gut check, then slowly reintroduce foods to see how you tolerate them. One week add dairy back, the next add grains, then nuts, etc.
- If you believe you have some sort of autoimmune condition or something is just not sitting well with your digestion, go get a food allergen blood test and eliminate what your body cannot tolerate to begin to heal your gut and see if that does not help. I would bet money that it will.
- Start drinking more water immediately. A gallon a day is honestly a great goal, but at least 2 liters is wonderful.
- Start listening to your body for when it craves what it needs. Eat when you are hungry, not because it is time. Eat until you are full, not until your plate is empty. Maybe you need a second plate.
- If your weight is not changing and you need to lose a few pounds, you might be overeating. I know stupid easy answer, right?
- Start with doable changes and tackle them one at a time. The quickest route to failure is establishing a routine that is not feasible within your current lifestyle. Overnight you are not going to be cooking every meal, fermenting your own foods, and brewing your own kombucha. That is okay!
- Start adding vegetables to every meal and eat those first.
- Start eating fruit for dessert if you usually have ice cream or something delightful.
- Start cooking at least four dinners at home a week. Then increase that number as you get into a routine.

- Start limiting alcohol. If you have wine every night, try to cut back to every other night and then eventually only on weekends.
- Start walking everywhere you can. Everywhere you can. It will become thoughtless and effortless fat loss over time.
- If you are serious and ready to go, start with the three-week gut check!

Your Guide to Your New Life

Everyday. Fill your plate with these first.

Staples: Clean healthy meats and fish. Veggies. Fruit. Tubers. Fermented foods.

If you are trying to lose weight, limit the fruit and tubers; eat them after a workout and earlier in the day.

Then maybe add these, almost everyday or a few days a week, depending on digestion.

Beans. Nuts. Peas. Lentils. Seeds. Preferably raw and pasture raised dairy.

Always cook your beans, peas, and lentils. Think about soaking and roasting your nuts if you have an adverse reaction. Enjoy raw dairy from a healthy cow if your body does well with milk! If not, try switching from cow to goat milk; if you still have trouble, omit entirely.

Maybes. A serving or two a day is plenty. See how you react, duh.

Quinoa. Rice. Oats.

I think a little quinoa and a little rice is totally fine. Quinoa you will get more bang for your buck, but see how you react to each. I also think some people need some oats in their life.

Opt for gluten free oats, and soak 'em overnight if you are concerned. (I personally soak them.) If you struggle with insulin resistance or blood sugar, I think it's a good idea to keep these aside most days as they carry a heavy glycemic load.

Now and again. When you are in the mood, do not overthink it and do not rely on it.

Dark chocolate. Treats. Alcohol. Processed carbs.

This is where you have to trust yourself. If you need something sweet or naughty, do it. Enjoy it, and then move on. The alcohol is tricky. Some people do great with a glass of red wine a night; some people abuse it.

You have to decide for yourself if it is helping you reach your goals or preventing them.

If a glass of wine a day keeps your heart warm, who am I to stand in the way of true love? Toe the line between enjoyment and indulgence.

Holding Yourself Accountable

The reality is you know deep in your bones if a food or a behavior is good for you. Listen to what your gut has to say about certain foods and even workouts.

For the most part, I know where my body is at when I am indulging too much or ignoring my nutrients. But sometimes, I need a little accountability. These are a few tools I use to keep myself on track without driving myself, and the hubs, insane.

Weighing In

I hate the scale with all my heart, but it really does help to keep me on track. My rule of thumb is to weight yourself no more than every two weeks. This will allow your body to work out bloat and water weight, and it will make sure that you are not suddenly a slave to the scale every morning.

Do not take that number too personally. Sometimes we carry extra water weight. Sometimes we really do have more muscle. Sometimes we had a minor indulgent weekend, and it shows up big time on the scale. There are millions of reasons for our fluctuations in weight. This is just a tool to keep yourself in the know of what is happening in your body, but it is NOT the answer.

Measurements

I personally do not measure myself, but it is a tool a lot of women find extremely helpful. I would use the same rule of thumb—every two weeks and no more.

Photos

Before and after photos are all the rage these days. For one they make you feel amazing when the after kicks the before's ass. But it really can be a powerful tool in assessing progress when that old scale can lie straight to your face.

So if you are up for before and afters, I would recommend taking a photo when you start your gut check, finish your gut check, and then on a MONTHLY basis take another picture, not every two weeks.
A good before and after photo has a solid front shot, back shot, and side shot. Don't want them on your phone? Me either. Email them to yourself and just make the subject line "before and after" so it is easy to search for later on.

Email them to ME if you want to share your glitter'd story with the world!

Must dos

- Avoid sugars and sweeteners (anything ended with an -ose), agave syrup
- Avoid natural raw sweeteners for the **first three weeks** such as honey and maple syrup
- Avoid all grains and breads forever preferably but for the first three weeks for sure
- Eat unlimited veggies, moderate fat and protein and limit carbs to 100 grams a day OR LESS preferably
- Incorporate a small amount of quinoa, wild rice, and sprouted whole grains AFTER the first three weeks to give your liver a chance to get rid of all stored glycogen and excess SUGAR
- Incorporate lower glycemic starchy vegetables like sweet potatoes, butternut squash, spaghetti squash a few times a week in place of processed carbs (breads, white stuff really)
- Avoid processed foods as MUCH as possible. In a wrapper? Processed.
- Drink. More. Water. Add slices of lemon, mint, cucumber, orange strawberries, blueberries, anything fruity and delightful!
- Limit fruit to 1-2 servings preferably eaten with protein or fat to slow the absorption of the sugars (1 serving = a handful or 1/4 cup)
- Eat when you're hungry, eat until your full and **do not worry about calories**. Worry about clean food choices.
- If you need a routine aim for eating 3 meals a day + 2 snacks + one nightly treat if needed

Treats

- Dark chocolate (couple pieces at night AFTER the first three weeks)
- Banana + almond butter
- Fruit for dessert at night with full-fat yogurt and cinnamon
- See treats recipe section

Supplements

- Ask your local health food store to recommend the most bio-available high quality brands and see resources for my favorite brands
- Fermented Cod liver / Butter Oil blend or Cod Liver oil capsules
- Calcium / Magnesium / Potassium (usually comes as a combo)
- Whey protein powder (I prefer organic grass-fed when possible, my favorite brand is Tera's Whey or Source organics, but choose a powder with the LEAST amount of ingredients and no artificial stuff)

A note on food prep

Be prepared to cook a lot of food twice a week. I like to cut on Sundays and Wednesdays. We will cook lots of chicken or beef to have for lunches and dinners. And I like to make a couple green sides to store ahead of time. I always have to have a good cooked protein on hand that I can heat up quickly after a long day of watching the Wubs and work. If I don't I tend to make a protein shake for dinner because I am so tired and just done for the day.

- Have cooked proteins and your favorite salad ingredients ready to go.
- Plan at least one day a week to prep food - Turn on some Italian or Mexican music and dance in the kitchen

My Typical Eats

To be honest, I tend to eat the same things over and over again. This makes prep easy.

	Option 1	Option 2	Option 3	Option 4
Breakfast	Buttered cup of Joe + Green Drink	2 eggs fried in coconut oil + bacon + greens	Crustless quiche	Gut healing porridge
Lunch	2 eggs fried in coconut oil + arugula salad dressed in balsamic / olive oil	Dinner leftovers from night before	Sausage + sauerkraut	Dinner leftovers from night before
Dinner	Pork chop + Salad	Buffalo chicken + sliced avocado + mixed greens salad	Taco salad	Breakfast for dinner! Two eggs + bacon + side of greens
Snacks	Coconut butter by the spoonful	Apple + Almond butter	Roll ups: Turkey deli meat + avocado slices + mustard	Proteinaccino
Treats	Kombucha in a wine glass	Paleo Fudge	Piece of dark chocolate	Glass of red wine

Tips on Buying

	Red meat + Fish	Poultry	Vegetables + Fruit + Herbs	Dairy	Fats (always choose organic)
Best	Organic + Pasture raised and 100% grass-fed Wild caught	Organic + Pasture raised	Organic + In season + Local	Raw + Organic + Always full fat	Coconut oil Raw butter Olive oil Palm oil Avocado oil Lard (grass-fed) Tallow (grass-fed) Fish oil Flax oil Avocados
Good	Grass-fed and finished or Organic with pasture access or Pasture raised	Just organic	Conventional Local + In season or Just organic	Organic Free range Pasture raised Minimally pasteurized	Nuts Seeds Flax oil
Avoid	Farmed fish Grain fed Cage raised Non-organic	Conventional raised	Conventional but no idea where it came from GMOs	Non-fat Added sugars Cage raised Non-organic	Trans-fats Hydrogenated oils Vegetable oils Non-organic raised animal fats

Grains limit to 2-3 servings a week	Dairy	Fats	Nuts	Herbs / Spices
Wild rice	Sour cream	Avocado Oil (good to cook with)	Almonds	Whatever your heart desires!
Quinoa	Cheese	Macadamia Oil (good to cook with)	Pecans	Just read the label, MSG sneaks its way into seasonings!
Sprouted grains and oats	Yogurt	Unprocessed Palm Oil (good to cook with)	Sunflower Seeds	
	Eggs	Butter/Ghee (pasture raised or grass fed) (good to cook with)	Brazil Nuts	
		Olive Oil (very low heat)	Pine Nuts	
		Walnut Oil (good to cook with)	Walnuts	
		Coconut Oil/Milk (good to cook with)	Hazelnuts	
		Sesame Oil (good to cook with)	Pistachios	
		Lard (grass-fed) + Tallow (grass-fed)	Derivative Butters	
		Flax oil	Hempseeds	
		Avocados	Pumpkin seeds	
			Macadamias	
			Sesame Seeds	

Veggies	Fruits - Preferred (limit to 1 - 2 servings a day)	Seafood	Meat
Avocados	Blackberries	Anchovies	Beef
Spinach	Boysenberries	Mahi Mahi	Goat
Jicama	Blueberries	Salmon	Pork
Celery	Cranberries	Bass	Chicken
Onions	Raspberries	Monkfish	Turkey
Tomatoes	Lemon	Sardines	Lamb
Leafy greens (any)	Lime	Cod	Bacon
Cauliflower	Pomegranate	Mullet	ANY wild game
Bell peppers	Coconut	Tilapia	
Shallots	Strawberries	Eel	
Beets	Orange	Tuna	
Kale	Tangerine	Haddock	
Cabbage	Grapes	Orange Roughy	
Bok choy	Goji Berries	Walleye	
Parsnips	Grapefruit	Halibut	
Zucchini	Other Fruits (limited servings, much higher sugar content)	Herring	
Squash	Apple (Green is best)	Red Snapper	
Cucumbers	Pears	Mackerel	
Broccoli	Apricot	Rockfish	
Carrots (limited 1-2 servings a day)	Kiwi	Abalone	
Yams (limited 1-2 servings a day)	Persimmon	Lobster	
Parsnips (limited 1-2 servings a day)	Banana (1/2 serving a day)	Scallops	
	Plums	Clams	
	Cherries	Mussels	
	Nectarine	Shrimp	
		Crab	
		Oysters	

8.
THREE
WEEK
GUT
CHECK

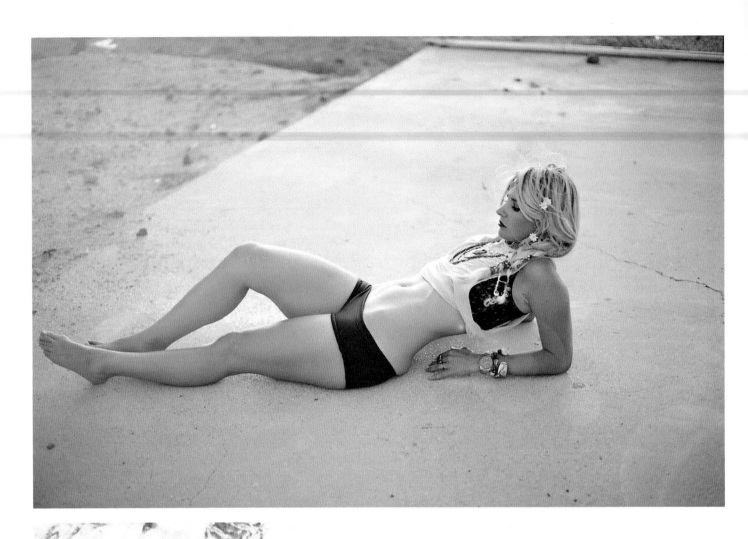

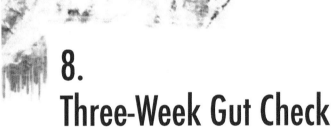

8.
Three-Week Gut Check

Time to get started!

Time to clean up your blood stream and start the process of healing your gut, reducing inflammation, and getting insulin under control!

I actually designed this three-week plan for my dad and me, who both suffer from achy joints, a not so healthy gut, and inflammation. He believes this gut check was life-changing. And it was, because he feels better.

Sure he lost weight, but he has less pain, and THAT is worth its weight in gold. I hit this gut check up anytime I am off track.

I highly recommend detoxing your body from all forms of sugar, alcohol, grains and processed foods for 21 days.

104

21 days is three weeks, sister. This is not because you need to lose weight; this is about hydrating and nourishing all the cells of your body in order to support healthy kidney, liver, and gut function.

This is also about trying to eliminate the source of inflammation in your body so you start to FEEL better inside and out.

- Eat the foods recommended.
- Drink a gallon of water every day.
- Move the way it feels good in your body, but don't kill yourself over it.
- Walk everywhere and use this time to honestly assess your health and well-being.
- For extra credit and ultra healing, make some good old fashioned bone broth and find a way to consume 8 ounces of it every day during the gut check. I personally am not a huge fan of drinking it warm in a mug, but some people LOVE it. I like to add a little coconut flour and make it into gravy to pour over my meats and veggies!

The Nerdy Deets

Why should you clean out your gut? Well, all disease starts in the gut, and many researchers and progressive doctors believe that what we call "diseases" are really just different forms of survival mechanisms for our body.

Before chronic disease comes systemic inflammation. But before systemic inflammation comes gut dysfunction. A permeable and damaged gut allows toxins to enter the body and cause havoc.

This three-week gut check is the BEGINNING of the road you shall travel to heal the gut and intestinal flora.

This gut check is comprised of three simple steps in three challenging but delightful weeks. This will not be the most exciting three weeks of your life. You will be challenged in ways you did not see possible. You will be changed in ways you did not see possible either.

After this gut check, don't over think your diet. Now is not the time to go nuts and shower and everything you could not have, now is the time to continue to enjoy feeling good in your skin. Keep eating good meats, veggies and fruits. Add dairy slowly and see how you digest it.

Add grains and nuts slowly, and again see how you digest them. When you're at a party, eat the cake. When you're at home, eat the veggies.

To be honest, gut healing can take MONTHS. So I encourage you to continue to avoid irritating foods like grains and sugars. At the very least, reintroduce these naughty foods one at a time and see how you react.

Or as previously discussed, go get a food allergen blood test and eliminate the foods you cannot handle. Because your gut suffers the most from food irritants.

Remove.
Nourish.
Supplement.

This is something I personally aim to do at least twice a year, sometimes more if something feels off. If I have a photo shoot or a big day coming up, you better believe this is my plan for three weeks.

If I go off the rails for a while, I come back to this for three intense weeks, and then I do so cyclically every twelve or so days I have some cheats for a few months.

::CAUTION::

This works well for someone who DOES NOT have severe acid reflux, GERD, or small intestine bacterial overgrowth (SIBO). One way to find out is to see how you feel after consuming fermented foods or probiotics. If they cause you some pretty miserable discomfort, you probably have a problem that needs attention greater than this three-week cleanse.

If you are already aware that you have acid reflux or GERD and/or SIBO, I direct you to Dr. Chris Kresser's site and urge you to seek help from a naturopath.

10 Tips to a Great Gut Check

1.   Wake up and drink a glass of water with half a lemon squeezed in it.
2.   Bonus points for drinking the **DETOX TEA** every morning, but good old fashioned green tea throughout the day is also fabulous.
3.   Drink up to a gallon of water a day. Squeeze fresh lemon in it when you can.
4.   Fill your plate with dark leafy greens and veggies you love. Try to get MOST of your plate full of greens!
5.   Eliminate coffee (at least for now) and if you must, replace it with green tea or matcha.
6.   Eliminate sugar (white, high fructose anything) and grains, (whole wheat, wheat, corn, kamut, barley)
7.   Avoid ALL dairy unless it is organic and raw, and/or organic full fat yogurt and you KNOW WITH 100% CERTAINTY THAT YOU ARE NOT DAIRY SENSITIVE. If you are unsure, skip it entirely.
8.   Avoid fruit except limited berries and lemons.
9.   Avoid all processed meats and farmed fish.
10.   Get rid of alcohol. Time to give your gut and your liver a break. No alcohol for three weeks. If you are used to a glass of wine every night, try pouring yourself a glass of kombucha in a wine glass instead.

Three-Week Gut Check

Step One. Remove irritating foods and toxins.

Remove this Shit

Foods

- Grains
- Sugar
- Conventional Meat
- GMOs (genetically modified foods)
- Processed foods (anything with a wrapper or box)
- Dairy (even organic/raw)
- If and ONLY if you have an **existing autoimmune condition**, remove all nightshade foods: tomatoes, eggplants, cocoa, coffee, peppers (black pepper is okay), tobacco, potatoes.

Toxins

- Tap water
- NSAIDs, antibiotics*
- Pesticides
- Harsh cleaning products

*Always consult a doctor, but remember that doctor probably will be against you stopping antibiotics. If this is the case, you need to don your white coat and start some research of your own.

Step Two. Nourish with good foods.

Nourish your Body

Water with lemon
One gallon a day. Fresh lemon squeezed in your water is best, and therapeutic grade lemon essential oil is the next best thing.

Ginger Spice Slice
Make ahead of time. Eat a slice before meals and/or throughout the day.
Ginger spice slice - Make ahead of time. Eat a slice before meals and/or throughout the day.

Bone broth and/or gelatin
As much as you can consume daily!

Fermented foods
Daily as much as you'd like! Sauerkraut, kimchi, kombucha, kefir, and full-fat pasture raised yogurt.

Green Tea
As much as you would like. So cleansing and great for your body!

Anti-inflammatory Omega-3 fats
Daily! Grass-fed beef, lamb, and wild caught fish

Coconut oil
Include 2 tablespoons daily either cooked with food, added to warm beverages, or served straight up if you can hack it.

Greens
As much as you would like. Go apeshit!
Herbals teas - I personally ADORE green tea, ginger, and chamomile.

Apple Cider Vinegar
Include 1-2 tablespoons daily! Shoot it straight up if you're gangster. Or add it to a big glass of water, or tea.

Three-Week Gut Check

Step three. Repair your gut with supplementation.

Supplement Your Gut

Supplements are entirely optional, but highly recommended to yield the full benefits of the gut flush.

L-glutamine
Daily

Magnesium Glycinate
Daily, usually at bedtime to help with rest!

Probiotic
Daily

Digestive Enzymes
Daily and before each meal

Aloe Vera Juice
1-2 ounces daily in the morning, icky, but good for the gut!

Three Week Gut Check

Foods to Enjoy and Nourish

See recipes for gut check approved creations!

Meat and Fish

- Meats – Grass-fed beef and lamb. Preferably organic, pasture-raised, and grass-fed. Check out www.eatwild.com for a state-by-state listing of organic and grass-fed animal products.
- Fish – Fresh or water-packed cold-water fish
- Wild game – Bison, elk, pheasant, rabbit, venison, etc.
- Poultry – Organic chicken, duck, organic turkey, free-range sugar-free turkey bacon

Vegetables

- Whole veggies, preferably organic and local
- Raw, steamed, sautéed, juiced, or roasted
- Honestly, if you need me to list out what's a vegetable, we have bigger fish to fry. Eat veggies; enjoy them. Just no white potatoes or corn. Please.

Fruit

- Only fresh and frozen berries, lemons, and limes
- Organic and local when possible, but berries should always be organic.

Alternative Dairys / Nut Milks

(unless you know of a nut allergy)
- Always unsweetened and free of xanthan gum
- Coconut milk, coconut water, coconut oil, coconut butter – unsweetened, no added flavor, organic when possible
- Hemp milk
- Nut milks – Almond milk, hazelnut milk

Eggs

(Unless you already know you cannot handle eggs or if you have an autoimmune condition, I would consider skipping eggs during the gut check.)

- Organic and pasture-raised eggs when possible
- Organic and free range is second best

Grains

(NO grains if you have an autoimmune condition)

- Limit to 1/4 cup a day, only if you really cannot live without them
- Quinoa
- Lentils

Other Shit

- Protein powders – Organic whey (preferably grass-fed) brown rice, hemp, or pea based, NO SOY!
- Go easy on nuts – Only a handful a day, and really I prefer them to be sprouted; if that's not possible, raw will do.
- No peanuts.
- Seeds – Chia seeds, hemp seeds, sesame seeds, sunflower seeds, etc.
- Nut and seed butters – Almond butter, cashew butter, tahini, etc. – unsweetened, unsalted, raw or dry-roasted, organic when possible BUT KEEP IT TO A MINIMUM.
- Nut and seed flours and meals – Almond flour, coconut flour, flax meal
- Bee pollen
- Spirulina, blue-green algae

Fats and Oils

- Look for organic expeller and cold-pressed, unrefined oils
- Oils - Almond oil, avocado oil, coconut oil, flax oil, extra-virgin olive oil, pumpkin oil, safflower oil, sesame oil, sunflower oil, walnut oil
- Avocados

Fermented/Probiotic Foods

- Sauerkraut
- Kimchi
- Kombucha
- Kefir
- Full-fat organic yogurt
- One glass of deep dark red wine a week

Drinks

- Mineral, filtered, and seltzer waters
- Yerba maté
- Coconut water
- Green juices
- Green and white teas
- Herbal teas

Sweeteners

- Whoa there, buttercup! ONLY a little bit like maybe once a day! MAYBE.
- Stevia
- Xylitol
- Monk fruit
- Honey (teaspoon or less per day)

Condiments and Pantry

- All herbs
- All spices
- Mustard
- Olives
- Sea salt
- Wheat-free tamari
- Vinegar
- Free-range or organic broth
- Capers
- Raw carob, raw chocolate/cacao (dairy- and sugar-free)
- Coconut liquid aminos
- Unsweetened ketchup
- Miso
- Nutritional yeast

Three Week Gut Check

Foods on the Naughty List

Avoid these for the next three weeks. You can do it.

Meat and fish
- Factory-farmed meats
- Processed meats – Canned meats, cold cuts, frankfurters/hot dogs
- Vegetable proteins

All Things Soy
- Tofu
- Soy milk
- Edamame
- Soy-based ice creams
- Soy sauce
- Soybean oil in processed foods

Beans
- Nuts and seeds
- Nuts that are roasted in oil
- Nut that have not been sprouted
- Peanuts
- Peanut butter

Fats and Oils
- Mayonnaise
- Salad dressings
- Spreads
- Butter
- Canola oil
- Margarine
- Processed oils
- Shortening

Vegetables
- Corn
- White potatoes
- Creamed vegetables

Fruit
All fruits except berries, lemon, and lime

Dairy
*If you have ever sensed that you do not do well with dairy, avoid for the first three weeks and then slowly introduce after to see how it feels. But always opt for **raw and organic** when possible. If you have any hormonal issues, dairy may not sit well with that.

- Any dairy that is not organic and raw
- Pasteurized / non-fat / sugar-added dairy
- Nondairy creamers

All grains
- All gluten-containing grains such as wheat, barley, rye, spelt
- All grains trying to not be named grains such as amaranth, buckwheat, kamut, millet, oats, rice—even if gluten-free

Drinks
- Alcohol
- Coffee (replace with green tea or Matcha if needed)
- Energy drinks
- Soda
- Fruit juice

Sweeteners
- All processed sugar
- Agave nectar, evaporated cane juice, honey, maple syrup
- Refined sugar – brown sugar, high-fructose corn syrup HFCS, white sugar
- Juice concentrates
- Splenda, Sweet'N Low, Equal, Sucralose

Condiments and Pantry
- Barbecue sauce
- Traditional soy sauce
- Teriyaki sauce
- Icky stuff like preservatives, artificial flavorings, dyes, MSG, thickeners

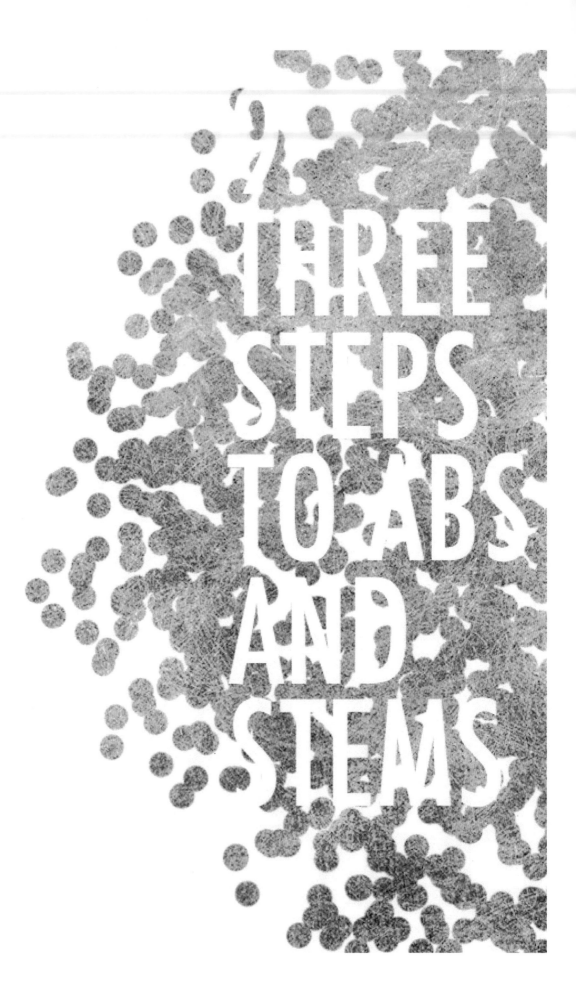

THREE STEPS TO ABS AND STEAMS

Sweat.

I refuse to serve a life sentenced
to the treadmill.

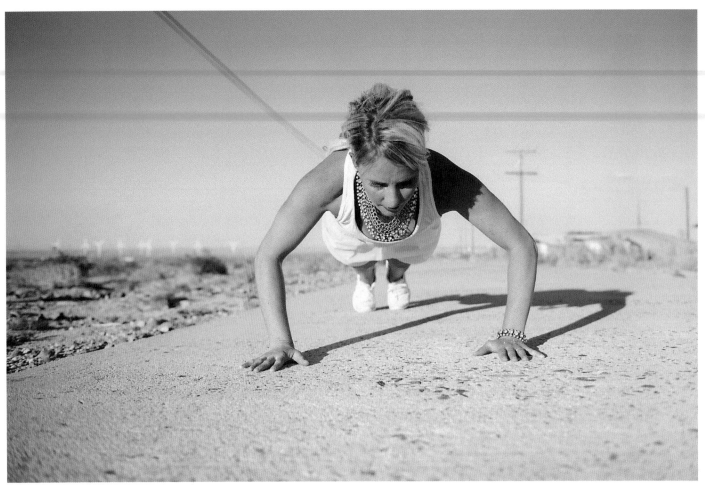

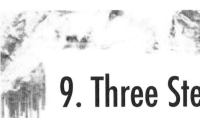

9. Three Steps to Stems and Abs

"Let's gossip to get our heart rates up."

- Carrie Bradshaw

Working out and keeping your body healthy is much simpler and easier than you would even like to believe. Ready for the million dollar secret to achieving the body you have always dreamed of?

Here it is in three Cliff Note worthy steps.

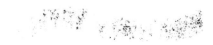

Step 1.
Nourish your body and your soul. Play. Sleep. Drink water.

Step 2.
Sprint your donk off once, MAYBE twice a week. Break up with counting cardio.

Step 3.
Challenge your muscles with your own body weight or some heavy shit a couple times a week.

116

The end. It really is and should be that simple. Will you be a supermodel in a month, no. But everything that is good for your body AND sustainable for a lifetime takes time and will work if you give it a chance.

Sustainable for a lifetime—that is the secret recipe to happiness and abs.

Smile and Move

Find something you enjoy doing, do it a few times a week every week, unless your body says it needs a break, and let it naturally fit into your schedule.

Don't force it.

Why, absolutely, you could kick your butt for twelve weeks, counting macros (all the food percentage of calories from carbs, protein, and fat), spending two hours a day in the gym, and you will likely achieve a body you never thought you could.

But you will lose it just as fast (if not faster) than you built it, because it is not sustainable over a lifetime. At least not in my house.

If you are a mother and a working mom and a wife trying to resemble somewhat of a smokin' haute human, please let me know how you have time for that shit, and I will personally send you a box of cookies because you is a beast, girlfriend!

Our Abusive Relationship with Fitness

Pour yourself a glass of kombucha in a dainty wine glass and let us toast to escaping our hamster wheel that is "health." Holler if you hear me on this. We think we have to eat carbs every few hours, or our blood sugar will drop and we will go into starvation mode.

Starvation mode will eat away our muscles AND store fat, so, shit, we need to eat more glucose in the form of any carb we can find.

BUT too much glucose from carbs will raise our insulin and start storing fat, so we have to spend hours and hours in the gym burning off the fat.

AND to workout a ton, we need lots of carbs for energy. SO basically, the only way we can actually be thin is to limit our calories as much as possible and work out until we collapse. Churn and burn, baby; binge and purge, churn and burn.

AND if you are working out regularly and intensely, eating healthy whole grain carbs on carbs on carbs, makes you ravenously hungry, constantly. We never get the right mix of nutrients in our mouths, so our bodies keep telling us we are hungry when we just crushed whole wheat pasta to get ready for our cardio marathon in the morning.

So here we are—still hungry, still chubby, and drenched in two hours worth of sweat.

We ladies believe cardio is the key to a smokin' haute bod, when actually it's strength training and intense but brief bursts of cardio. Excessive cardio combined with protein bars posing as food actually makes us store fat!

This yummy combo meal number 5 causes our bodies to eat away at muscle tissue for energy, which in turn slows our metabolism. We are hamsters on a treadmill. The road never ends, and our chub still rubs.

Having experienced a small bout of anorexia in my teens and learning that I could not outwork my diet or starve myself to be healthy was a tough lesson to learn. In the dark part of my soul, I remember how starving myself in my youth made me thinner, and this a dangerous mind frame to this day that I have to remind myself is wrong and simply will not work.

I do love my body with my whole heart, but I'd be lying to you and myself if I said I no longer had crazy moments of gazing in the mirror, finding an inch to pinch, and instantly thinking I need to skip dinner.
Luckily, my new self slaps my old teenage bitch self in the face, and I head out to crush bacon on days like this.

Move Happily. That's Enough.

Time to bitch slap the hamster wheel and start enjoying movement. Work out doing things you enjoy and that you will do each week. Unless your body says, *I don't want to move this week*, then LISTEN!

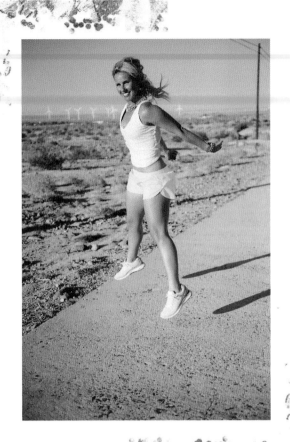

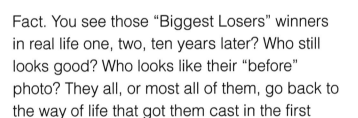

Fact. You see those "Biggest Losers" winners in real life one, two, ten years later? Who still looks good? Who looks like their "before" photo? They all, or most all of them, go back to the way of life that got them cast in the first place.

As MUCH as I adore and love Jillian Michaels and Bob Harper with my whole-est of hearts, the workouts they put them through on the ranch are never conducive to what they can, and will, do at home.

Should they have learned to make better choices? Absolutely. Were they set up to fail? Hmmmm, can't say.

When in your life have you had two to four hours a day to work out? Plus meal prep and make all of your meals from scratch? Ain't nobody got time for that. So what I propose is working out a few times a week, briefly, but kicking your ass in the few minutes you are moving and finding the joy in your movement.

How to Sweat Happily and Have Abs.

Step 1. Nourish body. Nourish soul. Go outside.

At this point, you should roll your eyes with annoyance because you've read the entire portion on clean eating and are ready to piss glitter. You heard me; you need nutrients, so why am I talking about nutrients in the sweat section? If you are not nourishing your body, you will not like looking at your body with the lights on. It is fact. Annoying but true, you cannot out sweat a bad diet, my friend.

Walk wherever and whenever you can and find joy every day. I know that is so hippy of me, but really, get out and go play. We live in a world that is tough, economically and emotionally speaking. We have to grind it out to make a living, so it is no wonder stress has become crippling.

When you can get outside and play, lather yourself in some coconut oil and lie in the sun for ten to twenty minutes a day. Vitamin D is your friend! Many doctors and scientists believe our lack of vitamin D actually is the cause of many of our current health ailments like cancer. Be smart with this, but seriously get some sun, girl.

Go for a hike, walk your dogs every night, take a family stroll—anything that is slow moving and not in front of your couch is a great idea for your body and mind. Think of our primal uncles again. They had to keep moving constantly at a very slow pace. Over time, this not only helps you burn fat, but it also keeps your bones, joints, and muscles strong.

Have you ever noticed how an older (and I mean older) person is seemingly healthy, but then has a fall or living arrangements are changed, making them less physically mobile; then six months later it's like they've aged ten years?

Keep moving (slowly) to keep moving. Park in the very last row at Costco and walk yourself to them samples. Go ahead and shower in those samples too! Free mother effing calories right there!

Step 2. Sleep.

Get your rest. Sleep, sleep, sleep (I cringe a little bit in writing this because as it stands it is currently 6:05 a.m., and I have been up for an hour and a half just so I can get work done before the rest of the family needs me to make them breakfast, wipe their butts, etc.).

But, for real, go to sleep earlier if you would like to shed more fat. By 10:30 p.m., I am a grumpy pumpkin.

Insufficient amounts of sleep can stimulate the release of ghrelin, an angry hormone that sends hunger signals and can decrease the regulation of leptin, which tells us that we are full and satisfied.

Basically, your body's natural energy system is trying to deal with the lack of recovery and rest you dealt it, so hormones start causing a ruckus just so you can function. As you know, once you piss those hormones off, they like to start storing fat just to prove a point.

They say abs are made in the kitchen. Agreed, but I'd say they're also made in the bedroom. Mmmkay, dirty bird, get your mind out of the gutter.

Yes, someone who is getting laid will be happier, which helps your body not hold onto stress and store fat, but I was talking about sleep.

Lack of slumber increases cortisol (think fat hormone), reduces testosterone production (think muscle hormone), and lowers muscle protein synthesis (think your actual building muscle tissue).

Finally, by not getting your body into slow wave sleep, the constructive stage of sleep where growth hormone secretion peaks, tissues never get a chance to heal, and muscles do not rebuild efficiently.

So get your snooze, missy.

Move slow. Get outside and play like a ten-year-old. Sleep. Wake up, and drink water.

Step 3. Build Muscle: Body Weight Workouts and My Philosophy with Strength Training

I believe females, and particularly female athletes, need to have great body awareness, control, and strength to perform and achieve the "toned" body we all lust for.

Body awareness and engaging your core for explosive movements not only translates to sport for increased performance, but it helps prevent injury in and out of sport and is an amazing way to burn fat.

The workout program I've created challenges your body in a proprioceptively rich environment, meaning your workouts take place in an unstable situation that causes the body to use its internal balance and stabilization to complete all movements safely.

The eff you just say? In English, you will use mostly your own body weight and CORE to challenge yourself in movement, and over time you will build more strength, overall balance, and learn how to use your core in all the movements your day requires.

Not to mention engaging a lot of muscles burns more energy, which translates to chub rubbing on.

I really love bodyweight workouts because these movements can be attacked anywhere, and even without supervision of a trainer, the chance of injury is much lower than swinging weights around by your lonesome. This is simply because you cannot progress faster than what your body will allow.

When you max out doing pushups, you max out doing pushups. You cannot jerk your body around to get one more rep in. You are just done. With weightlifting, you are tempted to progress faster than what your muscles are prepared for, and that is where injuries and workout ending pain start to happen.

Personally, I do mostly bodyweight workouts, and occasionally I will throw around a kettlebell. I think it stems from my arthritis, but weight workouts and my body are at odds with each other. Not to mention, I get big quickly lifting weights.

I know trainers everywhere want to kick me in the face, but I do not care; it is a fact.

Bodyweight workouts help me build lean muscle tissue. I also think "muscle memory" is real, and having squat and lifted a ton of weight in college for softball, my body is like, yeah, "Thunder thighs, let's fire up the old crew!" This is purely anecdotal evidence, but it does not mean it is not real. Take my word for what it is.

Not to mention I am super competitive. When I am lifting heavy weights, I tend to grit and rip it. For most of us who have never been properly taught how to use weights, this is a tremendous amount of pressure on not only our muscles, but on our joints and tendons.

Sometimes, I will add weight to squat or do some arms with a small amount of weight, but generally I kick my own donk with my own donk.

To make movements more difficult or to progress strength, I hold planks longer, add tiny jumps to movements, increase reps, and so forth.

When you put your body through intense workouts driven by your own weight, you teach your body how to balance itself. You teach your body how to react, move, jump, and stabilize in pressure situations. You teach your body to be a better athlete, and this helps your body stay healthy and thriving for life.

Now don't get it twisted, sister. I do think working out with weights can yield tremendous results for many individuals, but for me it brings pain and bulk. Bodyweight workouts are simply my jam.

In each strength session I have outlined, I ask the following:

Take each session to the point of volitional muscular fatigue. Basically, go until your muscles cannot go anymore. This will ensure that you have recruited and exhausted all muscle fibers, not just the first to fire. Use my reps and timers as suggestions, but when you are done, be done. When you are not done, challenge yourself with another round.
Add weights if it makes your heart warm and you need it!

Work in to your fullest capacity of energy and strength. I have created workouts that will challenge all different types of muscle fibers, and energy systems, so that your body composition changes quickly by pulling from fat storage and recruiting as many muscle fibers as possible. Move quickly, intensely, and, most importantly, safely through each exercise to burn the most.

Step 4. Sprint. Your. Ass. Off.

For the record, I hate traditional cardio. It takes forever, and in the long run can take a toll on the body. I believe adding HIIT training (high intensity interval training) and sprinting to your strength program is the real key to long-term health, fat loss, and increased performance in sports.

Interval training increases our exercise consumption post-workout, which means the body has to work harder to restore oxygen levels to a resting state. In essence, a shorter, more intense workout burns more calories over time and taps out your glycogen stores quickly (20.). So if you do an intense sprint workout in the morning and then follow it up with a long walk or walking about throughout your day, your body is more apt to pull from fat stores than glycogen.

Research also indicates that HIIT training completed just a couple times a week for a few rounds increases muscle mitochondrial capacity (meaning muscle energy and ability to grow) and helps to regulate blood sugar (21).

This is not a program where you will be grinding it out at the gym or the track for hours each week. No one has time for that, and your body certainly does not deserve that.

I believe the gym and traditional weights have an amazing place in our world to create healthier beings. But my personal philosophy is work your butt off—quickly, efficiently, where you can, when you can, and get on with it.

Step 5. Do it Your Way.

Some people hate lifting weights. Some people hate sprinting. Some people hate the gym. Some people hate sweat. If you are one of these peoples, dude, do it your way. I do believe you need to move your body, but if you hate sprinting, you will not do it every week. At least not well. If you hate the gym, you will not go much.

I am not here to turn you into a gym rat, I am here to say get off your ass, a few times a week for like thirty minutes.

Pilates? Yoga? Rock climbing? Barre Method? CrossFit? Walk? Hike? P90X? Rollerblade? Zumba? Ay ay ay ay ayyyyy!

Just move a few times a week.

Sometimes I am not into the gym, or lifting weights or doing bodyweight stuff. Some weeks I just want to run a few miles here and there. Awesome. Move and sweat happily, and stop being afraid of fitness.

Final Word Before Glimmering Some Sweat

If you have not exercised much in the past, you may not be ready for these movements. I suggest walking every day, jogging for ten to twenty minutes twice a week, and completing three sets of ten pushups, squats and lunges three times a week for four weeks before attempting this program.

Ready, set, Sweat!

x to the ohh, Whitters

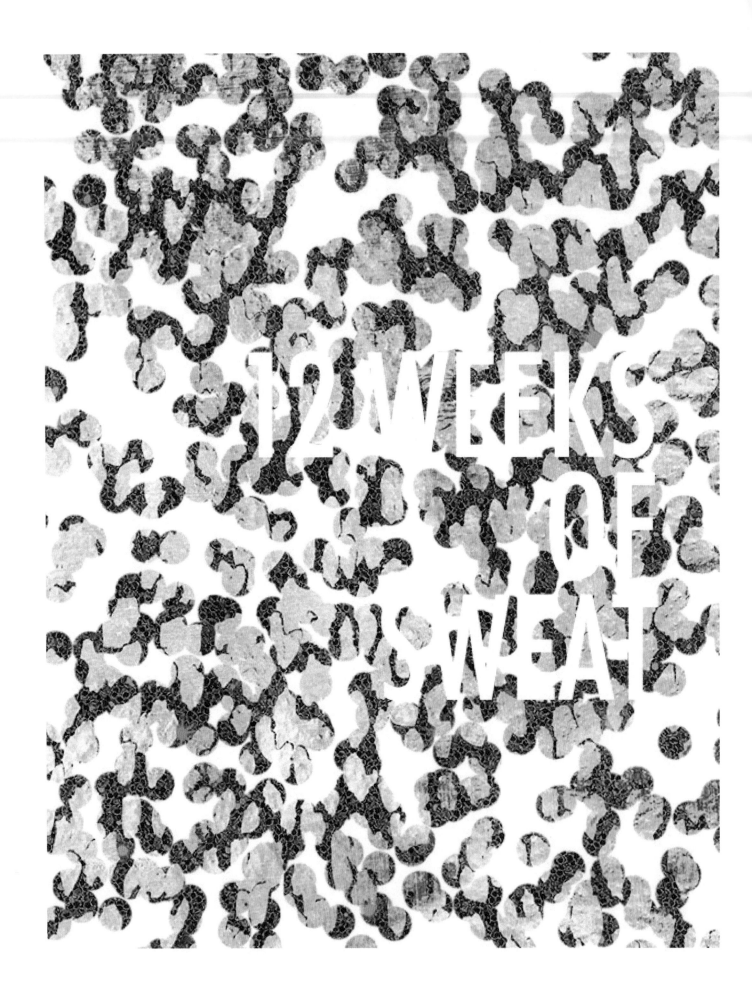

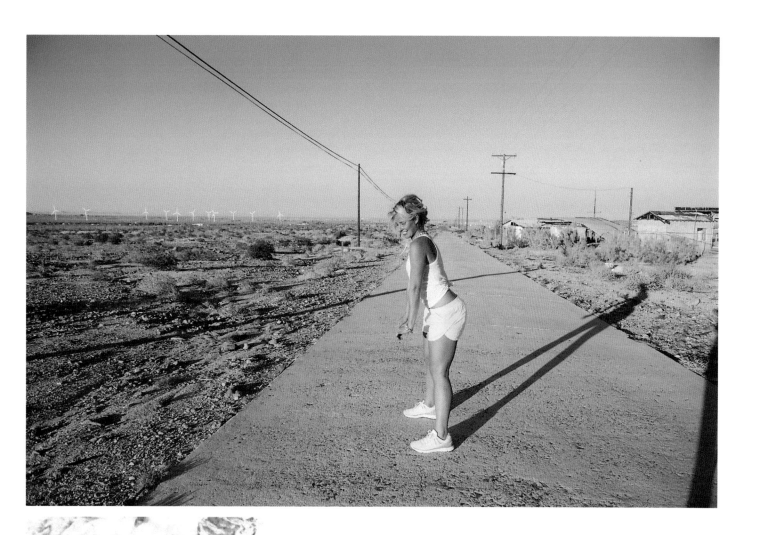

10. Workout Guide

Each week you will complete two **build** (bodyweight/strength) workouts, one **hiit that**(high intensity interval training) cardio session, and one **burn baby burn** session, which is a combination of fast paced cardio intervals and strength training.

How this works:

All training sessions can be completed from the comfort of your own living room, but I do suggest a private training session with a certified professional to learn any movements you are not familiar with.

Goddammit, Challenge Yourself and Be Smart

All movements are based off of your own bodyweight, but PLEASE add a set of dumbbells if you need some more oomph.

Always give your body the rest it needs when it needs it. The breakdown that follows works for me because I usually love to get one workout in a week at the gym on Sunday, and then I need to just squeeze in three or so workouts during my busy week.
So while I start my week of sweat on Sunday, you can start on Monday if you prefer. It's your life.

NO Reserving Energy

Each workout should take about 25 minutes AT THE VERY MOST. Some workouts may not "feel" they took long enough. But the goal is to WORK your heart out in each movement, sprint, or interval.

The next morning and probably two days after, you'll know you worked hard enough if you do the movements with intensity. When we work through intense exercises for long periods of time, we start to take our foot off the throttle because our body knows it needs to reserve energy.

Each session should make you want to fall down when you are done because you gave it absolutely EVERYTHING you have.

Each push-up, lunge, squat, or strength movement should be done with intensity, power, and focus. Each sprint should be the fastest you've ever run in your life, with good control, of course.

What about my days for cardio? Oh, girrrrll. We are actually breaking up with the elliptical.

Every workout will challenge your cardiovascular system whilst fighting your fat storage with muscle. Instead of worrying about logging minutes and calories on the elliptical, get outside and walk with the ones you love. Every day.

Sample Weekly Calendar

Now this is what works for me. Just like with your food, you will have to listen to your body when it comes to sweat equity. Please also adjust your workouts based on your personal schedule.

Sunday - build I (full body workout)
Monday - hiit that
Tuesday - foam roll / stretch / off
Wednesday – burn baby burn (or your own cardio)
Thursday - build II or haute housewife workout
Friday - foam roll / stretch / off
Saturday - play! sweat the way it makes you happy!

Where's the Cardio?

Great question. Cardio is optional as you will be working your cardiovascular system in every single workout you complete. That said, I do believe a little bit of steady-state cardio, in other words slow and easy cardio can be very beneficial. It is simply detrimental when that is ALL we do, and begin to abuse the treadmill. You will find me humming along running two or three miles pushing the BOB a couple times a week. AND you will see me walking every single day. Walking is the best form of cardio in my humble opinion. I actually find it meditative.

If you are a cardio queen or feel you need just a little more oomph in your weekly workouts, I say get two MAYBE three low intensity, steady state cardio in for 20-30 minutes. I like to complete my cardio before a build session, or replace a **burn baby burn** session with a short run.

All I ask is that you move happily, do not force yourself.

Tools

- Timer. I use my iPhone and the app Tabata Pro for most of my workouts. Gym Boss Trainer is also amazing. A good old fashioned stop watch works too, but I find the most success with the Tabata Pro app.
- Workout mat - Totally optional. I use the earth wherever I am, but you might be more comfortable with a sturdy workout mat.
- Jump rope - Also optional, but I believe a good jump rope makes for some good stems.
- Set of dumbbells - All of the workouts are based off of bodyweight, but you know the needs of your body better than I do. If you need to challenge yourself more in the strength movements, add your weights!
- Good friend - I think having a sweat partner in crime is an amazing way to enjoy workouts and hold yourself accountable. Totes optional, but definitely a good idea!

Sweaty Commandments

1. If you are unsure of how to complete a movement or workout sesh, please seek advice from a certified personal trainer.
2. If something hurts or just feels off, listen to your body and do not complete that movement or exercise.
3. If you need extra time to recover during a session, do it. These are suggestions. I would like you to push yourself and work as hard as you can in the moments you're moving, but you know your body better than I do. Be smart. Work hard.
4. Always warm up properly. I always prefer a five-minute jog or jump rope session to get my blood flowing.
5. Drink plenty of water. Drink more on days you sweat.
6. Foam roll once or twice a week, more if needed. This will help you with soreness, recovery, and bonus—it helps reduce cellulite!
7. Stretch lightly after each workout, and take time on your rest days to really stretch.
8. LISTEN to the needs of your body. Rest. If your body says no, don't force it because your calendar said you needed to move. Your muscles are much more intuitive than your calendar. Guaran-goddam-teed.
9. Incorporate the bonus haute housewife werkouts on days you feel like moving a bit; if you are truly sore or tired, let your muscles repair themselves.
10. Walk. Everywhere. Anywhere you can.

HAUTE HOUSEWIFE WORKOUT

This workout is great when you are traveling or are short on time but want to get your blood flowing. It's also a great complimentary workout to do when you just feel like you want a little bit more burn.

- Plie squats - 20
- Plank side to side dips - 20
- Plank leg raises - 20 (10 each leg)
- Donkey kicks - 20 (10 each leg)
- Side leg raises from knees - 20 (10 each leg)
- Booty bridge - 20
- Side to side sway in booty bridge - 20
- Repeat circuit 3 times

BUILD 1

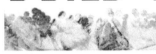

warm-up

- 2-5 minutes
- jump rope/jog

circuit

1. Jump squats - 15
2. Squats - 20
3. Inchworm plank walks - 10
4. Plank jacks - 20
5. Glute lunges - 20 (10 each leg)
6. Full sit-ups - 30

cool down

- Repeat circuit 4-5 times listen to your body as quickly but EFFICIENTLY as possible
- Be smart, once you feel your form start to break you are done
- Minimal rest if any
- Cool down - Jump rope, jog lightly or walk for 2-5 minutes

JUMP SQUATS X 15

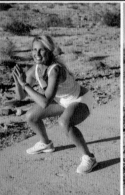 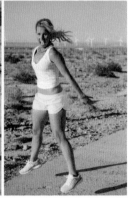

SQUATS X 20

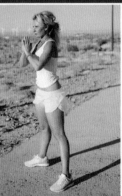 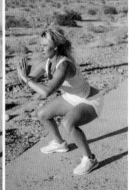

INCHWORMS X 10

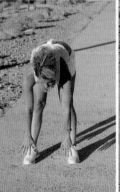 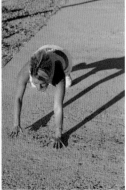

PLANK JACKS X 20

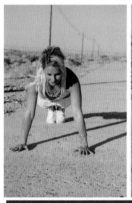 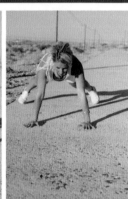

GLUTE LUNGE X 20

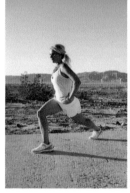 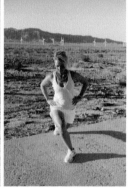

SITUPS X 30

please tell me you know how to do a full situp.

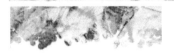

HIIT THAT

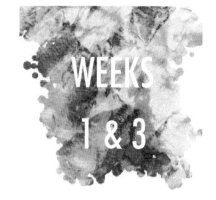

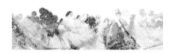

Warmup

Walk briskly or jog for 2-5 minutes

Move

- 30 second all out sprint
- 30 seconds rest
- Go for 10 sprints total
- Cool down - Jump rope, jog lightly or walk for 2-5 minutes!

**5 minutes may not "feel" like a long time, but the goal here is to sprint your heart out in each sprint. When we hold intense exercises for too long we start to take our foot off the throttle because our body knows it wants to reserve energy. NO reserving energy, each sprint should make you want to fall down. :)

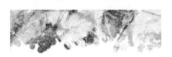

BUILD 2

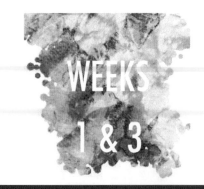

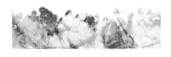

warm-up

- 2-5 minutes
- jump rope/jog

circuit

1. Jump lunges - 20
2. Pushups - 15
3. Dips - 20
4. Burpees - 10
5. Plank from elbows palms facing up - 30 seconds
6. Plank from hands - 30 seconds

cool down

- Repeat circuit 4-5 times listen to your body as quickly but EFFICIENTLY as possible
- Be smart, once you feel your form start to break you are done
- Cool down easy

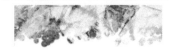

JUMP LUNGES X 20

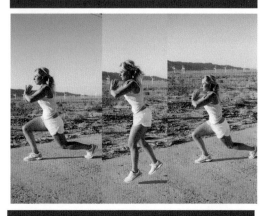

BURPEES X 10

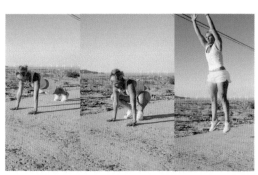

PUSHUPS X 15

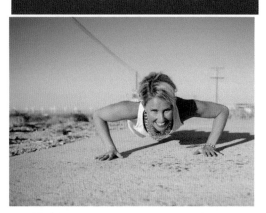

PLANK ELBOWS X 30

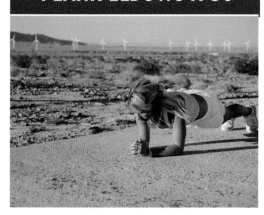

DIPS X 20

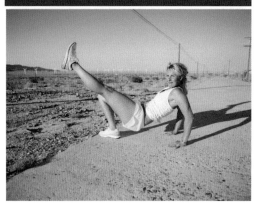

PLANK HANDS X 30 SECS

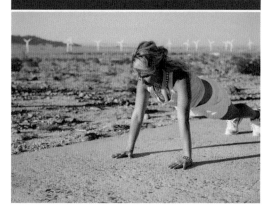

BURN BABY BURN

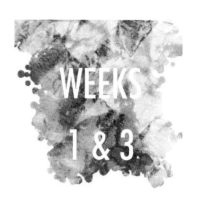

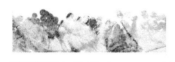

warm-up

- 2-5 minutes
- jump rope/jog

tabatas

1. Mountain climbers
2. Pushups
3. Plank jacks
4. Hindu squats

cool down

- Cool down - Jump rope, jog lightly or walk for 2-5 minutes

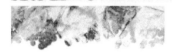

- This is a Tabata circuit where you work really hard for a short period of time, rest for a brief second and move to the next movement
- 20 seconds on each move get in as many reps as possible with GOOD form
- 10 seconds rest then move onto the next move
- Repeat circuit twice without stopping for 4 rounds total
- Easiest to set a Tabata Pro Timer App on iPhone for 8 rounds - 20 seconds work, 10 seconds rest

MOUNTAIN CLIMBERS

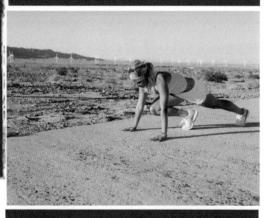

PLANK JACKS

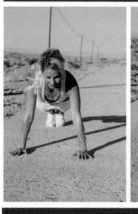
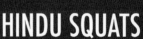

PUSHUPS

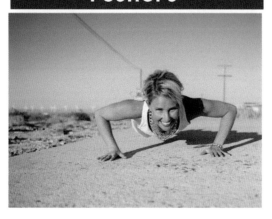

HINDU SQUATS

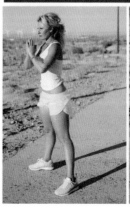
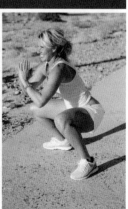

BUILD 1

WEEKS
2 & 4

warm-up

- 2-5 minutes
- jump rope/jog

circuit

1. High knees sprint in place w/ arms up high x 30 secs
2. Prisoner reverse lunges x 20
3. Prisoner squats x 20
4. Plie squats x 20
5. Plank jacks x 20
6. Side plank x 30 secs

cool down

- Repeat circuit 4-5 times listen to your body as quickly but EFFICIENTLY as possible
- Be smart, once you feel your form start to break you are done
- Minimal rest if any
- Cool down - Jump rope, jog lightly or walk for 2-5 minutes

HIGH KNEES SPRINT X 30

like, you lift your knees up as fast as you goddam can, arms straight up overhead.

PRISONER REV. LUNGE X 20

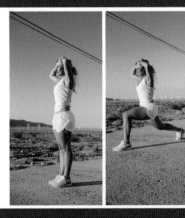

PRISONER SQUATS X 20

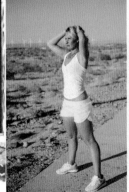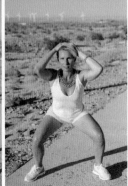

PLIE SQUATS X 30

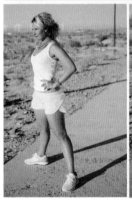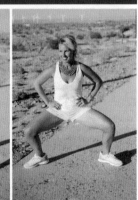

PLANK JACKS X 20

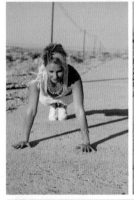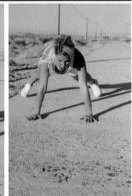

SIDE PLANK X 30 SECS

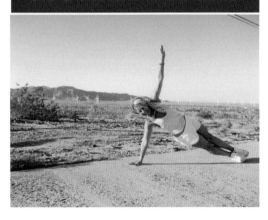

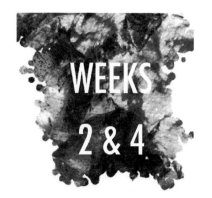

HIIT THAT

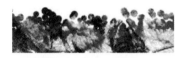

Warmup

Walk briskly or jog for 2-5 minutes

Hill-ups!
- 5 minute warm up walk or jog
- Find a good hill say 30 yards or 30 seconds to the top
- Sprint up the hill twice, walking down in between prints
- 20 pushups from toes or knees
- Repeat circuit for 5 rounds total
- 10 total sprints - 100 total pushups
- 90 seconds catch your breath walk
- 5 minutes walk

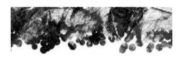

BUILD 2

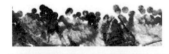

warm-up

- 2-5 minutes
- jump rope/jog

circuit

1. Burpees x 15
2. Offset pushups x 15
3. Dips x 20
4. 50 meter sprint or 30 secs sprint in place!
5. Tummy tucks x 20
6. Plank from elbows x 45 secs

cool down

- Repeat circuit 4-5 times listen to your body as quickly but EFFICIENTLY as possible
- Be smart, once you feel your form start to break you are done
- Minimal rest if any
- Cool down - Jump rope, jog lightly or walk for 2-5 minutes

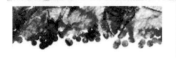

BURPEES X 15

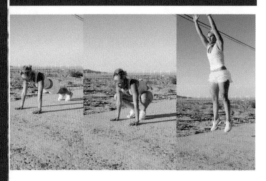

SPRINT!

Sprint your mother effing ass off right now. Outside. In your living room. Just go.

OFFSET PUSHUPS X 15

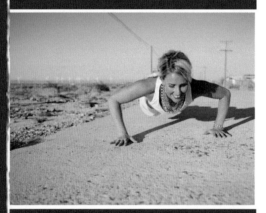

TUMMY TUCKS X 20

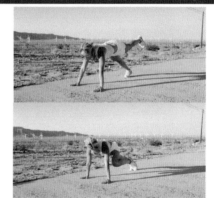

DIPS X 20

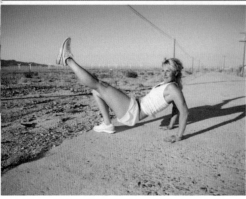

PLANK X 45 SECS

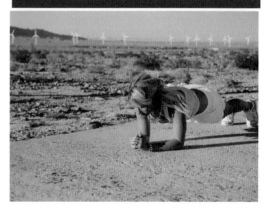

BURN BABY BURN

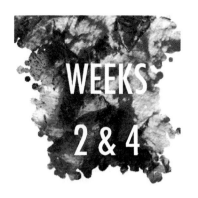

WEEKS 2 & 4

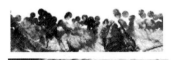

warm-up

- 2-5 minutes
- jump rope/jog

tabatas

1. Plie squat hops
2. Diamond pushups
3. Prisoner reverse lunges
4. Jump squats

cool down

- Cool down - Jump rope, jog lightly or walk for 2-5 minutes

- This is a Tabata circuit where you work really hard for a short period of time, rest for a brief second and move to the next movement
- 20 seconds on each move get in as many reps as possible with GOOD form
- 10 seconds rest then move onto the next move
- Repeat circuit twice without stopping for 4 rounds total
- Easiest to set a Tabata Pro Timer App on iPhone for 8 rounds - 20 seconds work, 10 seconds rest

PLIE SQUAT HOPS

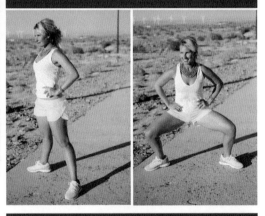

PRISONER REV LUNGE

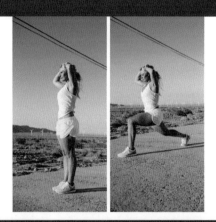
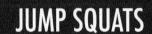

DIAMOND PUSHUPS

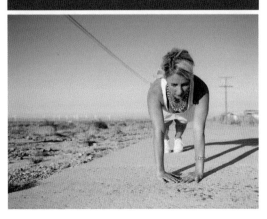

JUMP SQUATS

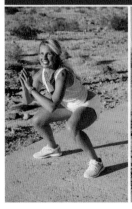
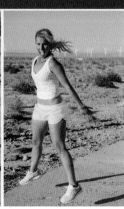

BUILD 1

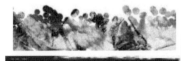

warm-up
- 2-5 minutes
- jump rope/jog

circuit
1. Line drive side to side hops - 20
2. Prisoner squats - 15
3. Side lunge to punish pulse - 20 (10 lunges + 10 pulses each leg)
4. Step ups - 20
5. Jump rope - 1 minute
6. Plank + hip dips side to side - 1 minute

cool down
- Repeat circuit 4-5 times listen to your body as quickly but EFFICIENTLY as possible
- Be smart, once you feel your form start to break you are done
- Minimal rest if any
- Cool down - Jump rope, jog lightly or walk

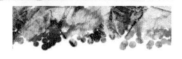

LINE DRIVE HOPS x 20

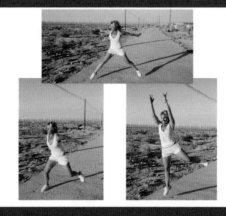

PRISONER SQUATS x 15

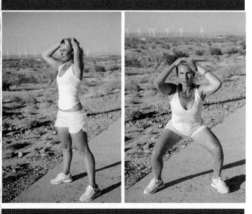

SIDE LUNGE TO PULSE x 20

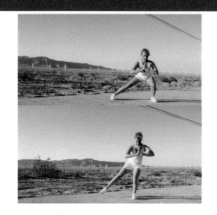

STEP UPS x 20

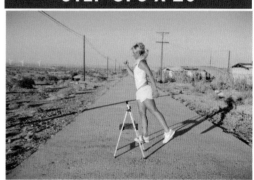

JUMP ROPE x 1 min

jump rope. or pretend like you have one.

PLANK + HIP DIPS x 1 min

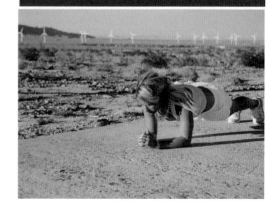

HIIT THAT

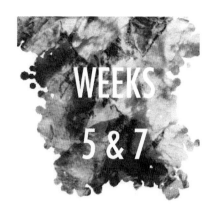

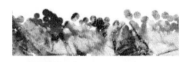

Warmup

Walk briskly or jog for 2-5 minutes

All out sprint!

- 20 seconds on - 10 seconds rest
- Repeat for 8 sprints total
- 90 seconds rest and recover
- Repeat for 8 more sprints
- Walk or jog for 2-5 minutes, stretch easy and recover

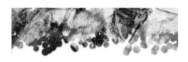

BUILD 2

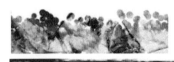

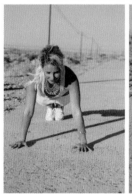 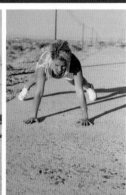

WEEKS 5 & 7

warm-up
- 2-5 minutes
- jump rope/jog

circuit

1. Jump rope - 1 minute
2. Wide-leg pushups - 20
3. Dips - 20
4. Mountain climbers - 1 minute
5. Plank from hands - 1 minute
6. Sit-ups - 30

cool down
- Repeat circuit 4-5 times listen to your body as quickly but EFFICIENTLY as possible
- Be smart, once you feel your form start to break you are done
- Minimal rest if any
- Cool down - Jump rope, jog lightly or walk for

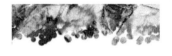

JUMP ROPE X 1 MIN

jump rope.
or pretend like
you have one.

MOUNTAIN CLIMBERS X 1 MIN

WIDE LEG PUSHUPS X 20

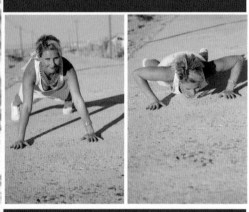

PLANK X 1 MIN

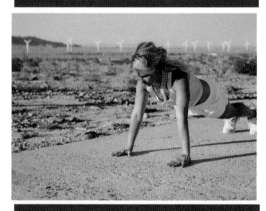

DIPS X 20

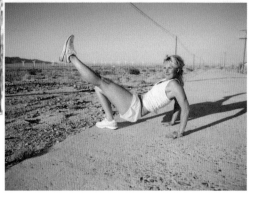

SITUPS X 30

please tell me
you know
how to do a
full situp.

BURN BABY BURN

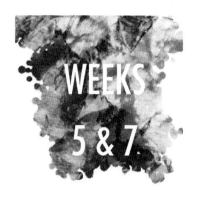

WEEKS 5 & 7

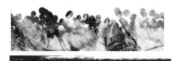

warm-up

- 2-5 minutes
- jump rope/jog

tabatas

1. Seal jacks
2. Prisoner reverse lunges
3. Burpees
4. Crab side walks (switch directions each set)

cool down

- Cool down - Jump rope, jog lightly or walk for 2-5 minutes

- This is a Tabata circuit where you work really hard for a short period of time, rest for a brief second and move to the next movement
- 20 seconds on each move get in as many reps as possible with GOOD form
- 10 seconds rest then move onto the next move
- Repeat circuit twice without stopping for 4 rounds total
- Easiest to set a Tabata Pro Timer App on iPhone for 8 rounds - 20 seconds work, 10 seconds rest

SEAL JACKS

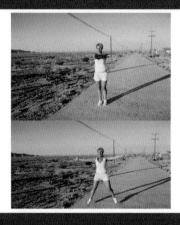

BURPEES

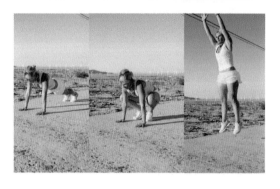

PRISONER LUNGES

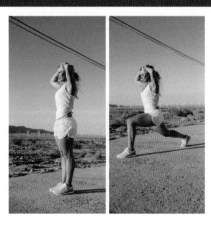

CRAB SIDE WALKS

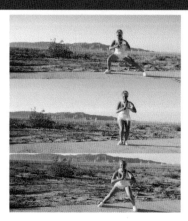

BUILD 1

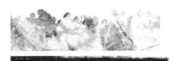

warm-up
- 2-5 minutes
- jump rope/jog

circuit
1. X jumps - 20
2. Pushups - 20
3. Prisoner squats - 30
4. Glute lunges - 30
5. Plie squats - 30
6. Row your boats - 30

cool down
- Repeat circuit 4-5 times listen to your body as quickly but EFFICIENTLY as possible
- Be smart, once you feel your form start to break you are done
- Minimal rest if any
- Cool down - Jump rope, jog lightly or walk for 2-5 minutes

X JUMPS X 20
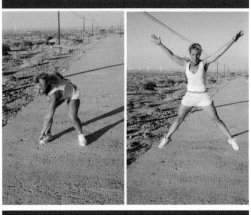

GLUTE LUNGES X 30
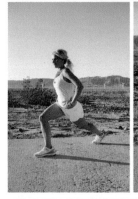
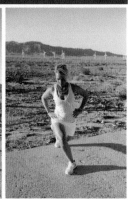

PUSHUPS X 20
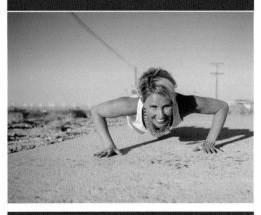

PLIE SQUATS X 30
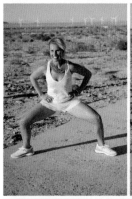
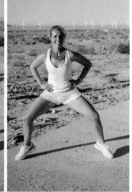

PRISONER SQUATS X 30
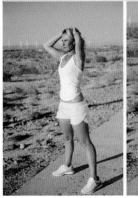
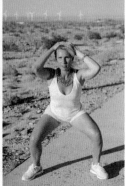

ROW YOUR BOATS X 30
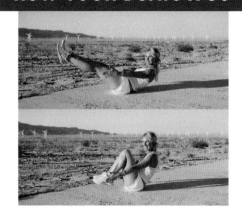

HIIT THAT

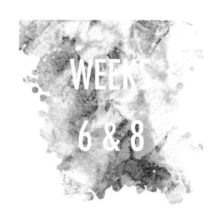

Warmup

Walk briskly or jog for 2-5 minutes

Earn your sprints!
1. Wide grip pushups - 20
2. Row your boats - 20
3. Prisoner lunges - 30
4. Mountain climbers - 20
5. 40 seconds shuttle sprint or straight sprint (Set a timer and find a short distance and sprint back and forth until 40 seconds is up.)
- Repeat for 4 rounds total! No rest.

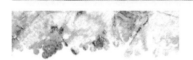

BUILD 2

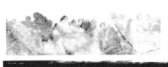

warm-up

- 2-5 minutes
- jump rope/jog

circuit

1. Star jumps - 15
2. Inchworm planks - 20
3. One leg lunge hops - 30
4. Diamond pushups - 15
5. Mountain climbers - 1 minute
6. Plank from hands - 1 minute

cool down

- Repeat circuit 4-5 times listen to your body as quickly but EFFICIENTLY as possible
- Be smart, once you feel your form start to break you are done
- Minimal rest if any
- Cool down - Jump rope, jog lightly or walk for 2-5

STAR JUMPS X 15

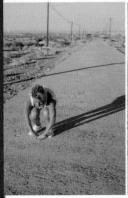
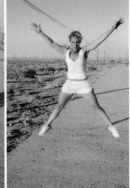

INCHWORMS X 20

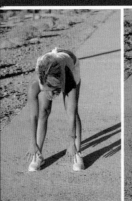
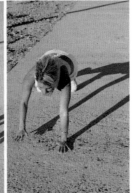

ONE LEG LUNGE HOPS X 30

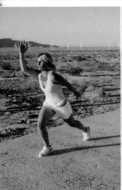
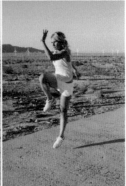

DIAMOND PUSHUPS X 15

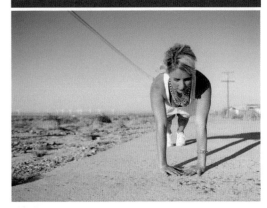

MOUNTAIN CLIMBERS X 1 MIN

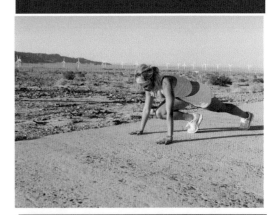

PLANK X 1 MIN

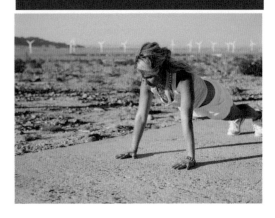

BURN BABY BURN

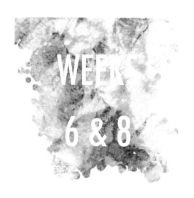

warm-up

- 2-5 minutes
- jump rope/jog

tabatas

1. Burpees
2. Walking pushups (pushup walk hands left, pushup walk hand right)
3. Cross-body mountain climbers
4. Walking plank

cool down

- This is a Tabata circuit where you work really hard for a short period of time, rest for a brief second and move to the next movement
- 20 seconds on each move get in as many reps as possible with GOOD form
- 10 seconds rest then move onto the next move
- Repeat circuit twice without stopping for 4 rounds total
- Easiest to set a Tabata Pro Timer App on iPhone for 8 rounds
  - 20 seconds work, 10 seconds rest

BURPEES

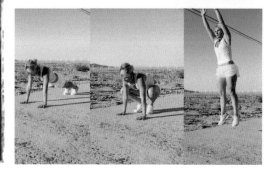

CROSS MOUNTAIN

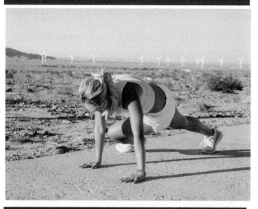

WALKING PUSHUPS

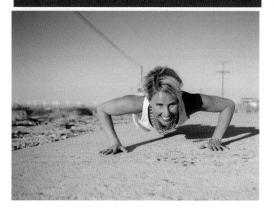

WALKING PLANK

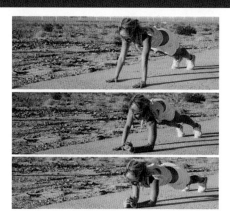

BUILD 1

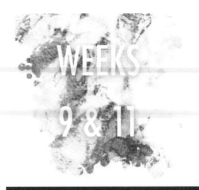

warm-up
- 2-5 minutes
- jump rope/jog

circuit
1. Squat thrusts - 30
2. Diamond pushups - 20
3. Dips - 30
4. Star jumps - 20
5. Step ups - 30 (use a bench or box)
6. Full situps - 30

cool down
- Repeat circuit 4-5 times listen to your body as quickly but EFFICIENTLY as possible
- Be smart, once you feel your form start to break you are done
- Minimal rest if any
- Cool down - Jump rope, jog lightly or walk for 2-5 minutes

SQUAT THRUSTS X 30

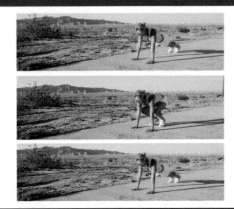

STAR JUMPS X 20

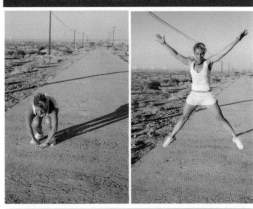

DIAMOND PUSHUPS X 20

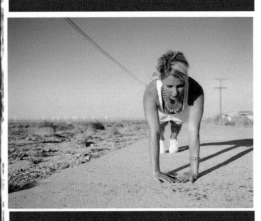

STEP UPS X 20

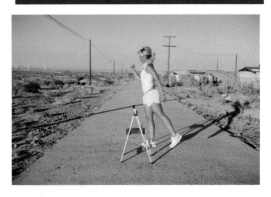

DIPS X 30

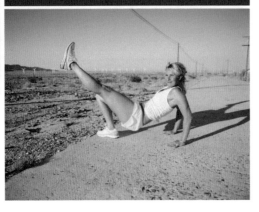

SITUPS X 30

please tell me you know how to do a full situp.

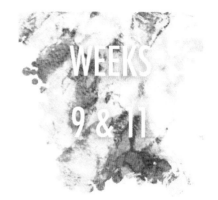

HIIT THAT

Warmup

Walk briskly or jog for 2-5 minutes

Toot it, boot it, sprint it

1. Walk or jog 5 minutes
2. Diamond pushups - 20
3. Squats - 30
4. Tummy tucks - 30
5. Off Set Pushup: 5 reps each side
6. Sprint - 1 minute - 100 yards or so
7. Rest ONLY when needed and complete for 4 total rounds
8. Walk for 5 minutes

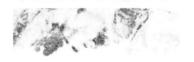

BUILD 2

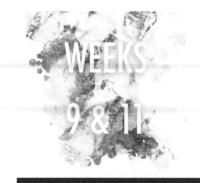

warm-up
- 2-5 minutes
- jump rope/jog

circuit

1. Sumo squat jumps - 20
2. Side plank - 1 minute (switch sides each set)
3. Plank from elbows - 1 minute
4. Plie squat hops - 30
5. Line drive hops - 20
6. Pushups to failure - As many reps as you can until your form breaks

cool down
- Repeat circuit 4-5 times listen to your body as quickly but EFFICIENTLY as possible
- Be smart, once you feel your form start to break you are done

SUMO SQUAT JUMPS X

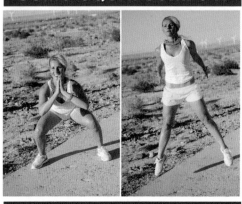

SIDE PLANK X 1 MIN

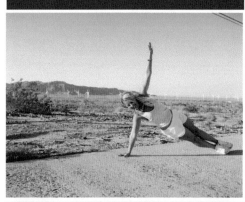

PLANK X 1 MIN

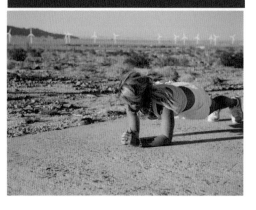

PLIE SQUAT HOPS X 30

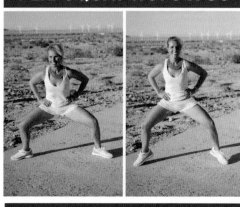

LINE DRIVE HOPS X 20

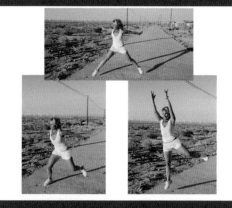

PUSHUPS TO FAILURE

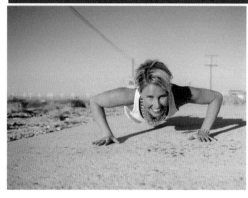

BURN BABY BURN

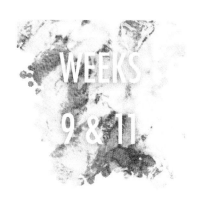
- This is a Tabata circuit where you work really hard for a short period of time, rest for a brief second and move to the next movement
- 20 seconds on each move get in as many reps as possible with GOOD form
- 10 seconds rest then move onto the next move
- Repeat circuit twice without stopping for 4 rounds total
- Easiest to set a Tabata Pro Timer App on iPhone for 8 rounds - 20 seconds work, 10 seconds rest

warm-up
- 2-5 minutes
- jump rope/jog

tabatas

1. Burpees
2. Dips w/ alternating legs
3. Cross-body mountain climbers
4. Plie squat jumps

cool down
- Cool down - Jump rope, jog lightly or walk for 2-5

BURPEES
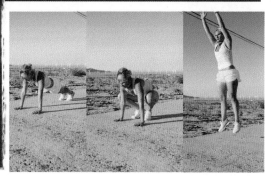

CROSS MOUNTAIN
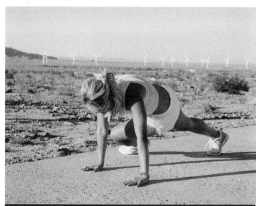

DIPS W/ LEGS
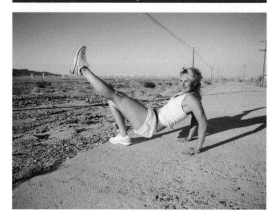

PLIE SQUAT JUMPS
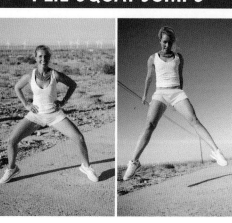

BUILD 1

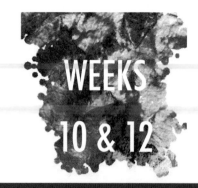

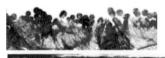

warm-up
- 2-5 minutes
- jump rope/jog

circuit
1. Burpees - 20
2. Wide leg pushups - 20
3. Sumo squat + leg lifts - 30
4. Glute lunges - 30
5. Jump lunges - 20
6. Myoatic crunches - 15

cool down
- Repeat circuit 4-5 times listen to your body as quickly but EFFICIENTLY as possible
- Be smart, once you feel your form start to break you are done
- Minimal rest if any
- Cool down - Jump rope, jog lightly or walk for 2-5

BURPEES X 20
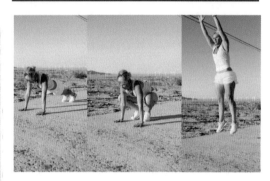

WIDE LEG PUSHUPS X 20
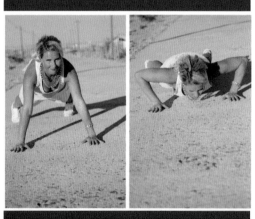

SUMO + LEG LIFT X 30
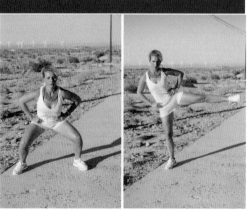

GLUTE LUNGES X 30
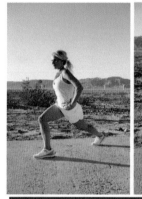
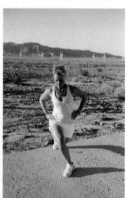

JUMP LUNGES X 20
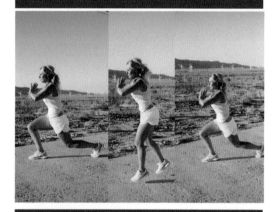

MYOATIC CRUNCHES X 15
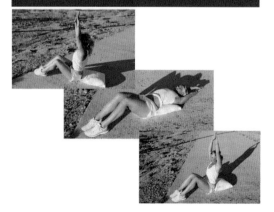

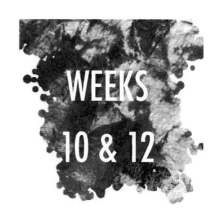

HIIT THAT

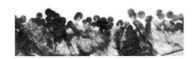

Warmup

Walk briskly or jog for 2-5 minutes

7 deadly sprints

1. Walk or jog for 5 minutes
2. Sprint - 50 yards or 45 seconds
3. Pushups - 7 reps
4. Squat Jumps - 7 reps
5. Burpees - 7 reps
6. Squat thrusts- 7
- Repeat 7 full rounds resting ONLY when needed!
- Walk for 5 minutes

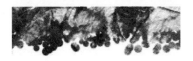

BUILD 2

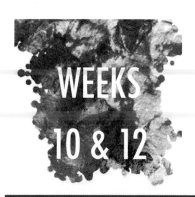

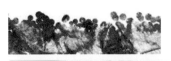

warm-up

- 2-5 minutes
- jump rope/jog

circuit

1. Star jumps - 20
2. Broken plank - 1 min
3. Dead lifts + pulses - 30 - (10 dead lifts + 5 pulses x 3 times)
4. Wide leg pushups - 20
5. Step ups - 30
6. Dips - 30

cool down

- Repeat circuit 4-5 times listen to your body as quickly but EFFICIENTLY as possible
- Be smart, once you feel your form start to break you are done
- Minimal rest if any
- Cool down - Jump rope, jog lightly or walk for 2-5 minutes

STAR JUMPS X 20

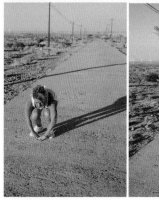
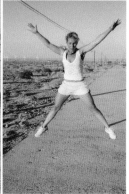

WIDE LEG PUSHUPS X 20

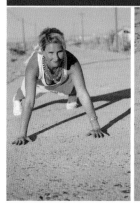
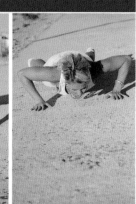

BROKEN PLANK X 1 MIN

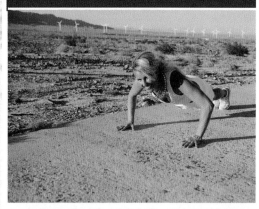

STEP UPS X 30

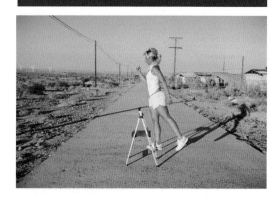

DEAD LIFTS TO PULSE x 30

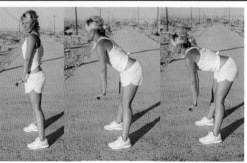

DIPS X 30

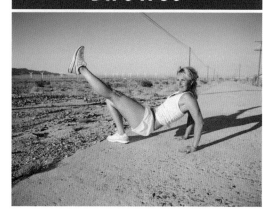

BURN BABY BURN

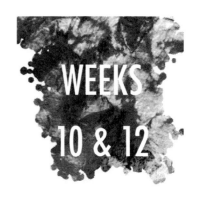

WEEKS 10 & 12

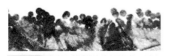

warm-up
- 2-5 minutes
- jump rope/jog

tabatas
1. X jumps
2. Side lunge to punish pulse (switch legs each set)
3. Cross-body mountain climbers
4. Wide grip

cool down
- Cool down - Jump rope, jog lightly or walk for 2-5 minutes

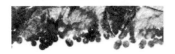

- This is a Tabata circuit where you work really hard for a short period of time, rest for a brief second and move to the next movement
- 20 seconds on each move get in as many reps as possible with GOOD form
- 10 seconds rest then move onto the next move
- Repeat circuit twice without stopping for 4 rounds total
- Easiest to set a Tabata Pro Timer App on iPhone for 8 rounds - 20 seconds work, 10 seconds rest

X JUMPS

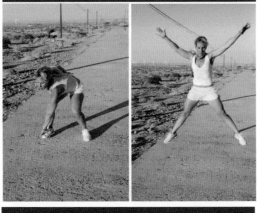

CROSS MOUNTAIN

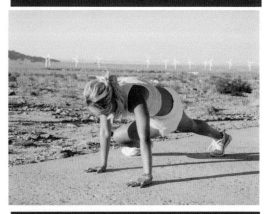

SIDE LUNGE TO PULSE

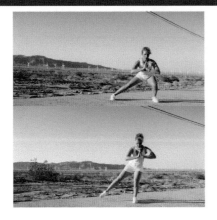

WIDE GRIP PUSHUPS

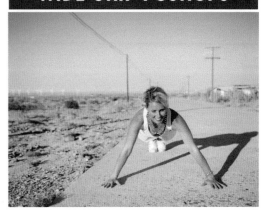

P.S. If you complete a workout, snap a photo and tag me on the Instagram machine for a shoutout!

@eatcleanpissglitter

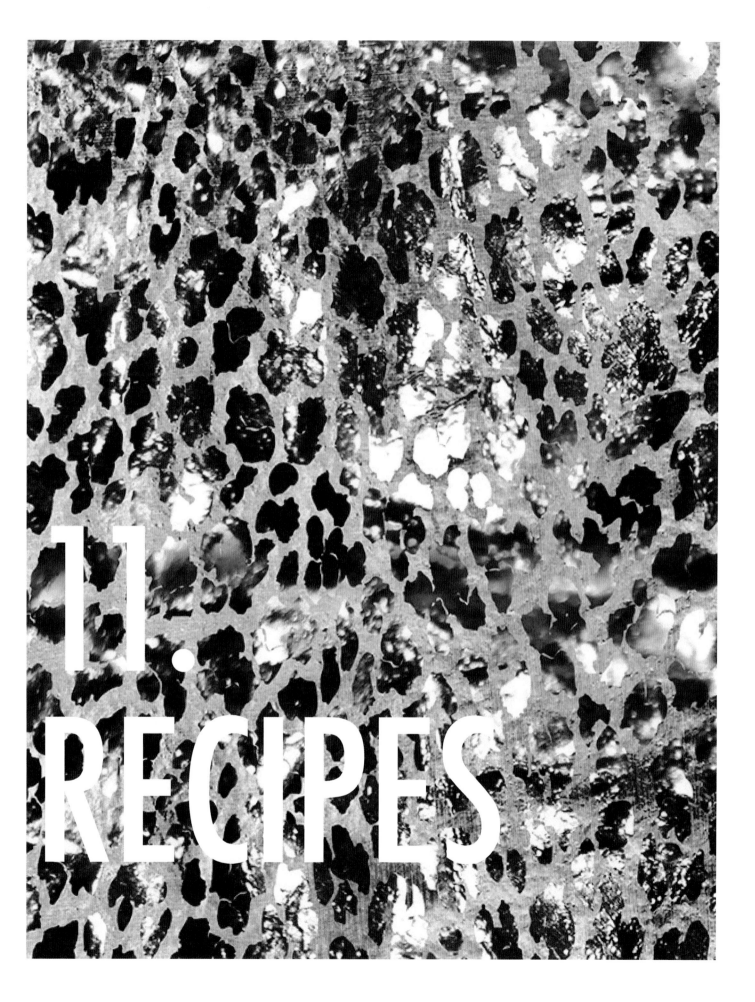

11.
RECIPES

RECIPES

Basic build a meal

- 4 - 8 ounces of meat or fish of choice
- Unlimited veggies (corn limited to twice a week)
- Fats – olive oil, coconut oil, avocado oil, nuts of choice, full fat cheese, grass-fed butter, ghee

Breakfast

Buttered Cup of Joe

- 1 cup of coffee however you like it made (preferably low toxin, organic if possible)
- 1 tablespoon of coconut oil
- 1 tablespoon of high quality butter or ghee
- 1/2 teaspoon of cinnamon
- 1/4 teaspoon of sea salt
- 1/2 teaspoon of high quality vanilla
- Option to add 1 tablespoon of grass-fed gelatin
- Blend everything for two minutes. Top with cinnamon and a little sea salt. Slurp. Good morning!

Egg Breakfasts

- 2 - 3 eggs cooked any style in coconut oil or grass-fed butter (Kerrygold brand available at Trader Joe's, Whole Foods, Sprouts and Cosco)
- 2 - 3 pieces of organic sausage or bacon (check package to make sure it is not cured in sugar)
- Any veggies you like, spices, hot sauce, seasonings
- 1/2 grapefruit or 1/4 cup of berries (optional)
- 1/4 avocado (optional)

Chocolate Morning Shake

- 1 cup unsweetened almond milk or water or coconut milk
- 1 serving of protein powder of choice (I prefer Tera's Whey or Source Organics Grass- Fed Whey)
- 1 tbsp organic heavy whipping cream (yes you read that right)
- 2 tbsp almond butter
- 1/4 banana
- 1/4 cup of ice

Mexican Mocha Shake

- One cup of freshly brewed coffee preferably chilled
- Scoop of your favorite high quality chocolate whey powder
- 1 tablespoon of unsweetened cocoa powder
- 2 shakes of cayenne
- 1/4 teaspoon of cinnamon
- Dash of stevia (optional)
- Blend with 5 or so ice cubes
- Top with cinnamon and a little sea salt for a caramel-y delight

Wubba's Weekly Crustless Quiche

- 6 eggs
- 1 cup of organic raw milk
- Meat of choice - I like to add a few chopped up pieces of previously cooked bacon, or sliced breakfast sausage
- 2 or so tablespoons of high quality cheese - I love Kerrygold
- Veggies of choice - I like chopped spinach and tomatoes
- 1 tablespoon grass-fed gelatin (optional) add to eggs and let sit one minute
- Beat eggs and milk together. Then add 1 tablespoon of optional gelatin. Add meat and veggies. Grease 8-9 inch pie pan with coconut oil or butter, and cook at 350 for about 25 minutes depending on your oven

Breakfast Cake

- 3 eggs beat well
- 1 tablespoon grass-fed gelatin (optional) add to eggs and let sit one minute
- 4 tablespoons cocoa powder
- 1 cup raw milk
- 1/4 cup flax meal
- 1/4 cup protein powder
- 1/4 cup hemp seeds
- 1/4 cup of berries
- 2 tablespoons roasted nut butter
- Stevia or a tablespoon of raw honey to sweeten
- Beat eggs, add gelatin let sit for one minute.
- Top with 1/4 cup of full fat yogurt mixed with stevia melted on the stove and drizzled over

Overnight Slow Cooker Oatmeal

You want to soak your oats in some sort of acid medium that will destroy the phytic acid and make them digestible. I usually begin prep the day before to give the oats enough soaking time (for example place all ingredients in your slow cooker on Sunday morning (or Saturday night) for a Monday morning breakfast).

- 1 cup Irish steel cut oats
- 2 tablespoons whey, yogurt, kefir, buttermilk, lemon juice, or vinegar
- 4 cups warm water
- 1/2 teaspoon sea salt
- butter, coconut oil, and/or cream
- optional toppings – natural sweetener, chopped nuts, dried fruit, shredded coconut, freshly ground flax seeds

1. Place oats, whey (or other acid medium), and warm water in the insert of your slow cooker and let soak for 12 hours.
2. The night before you want to serve the oatmeal (or 8-12 hours before) turn the slow cooker on to low.
3. Before serving, stir in sea salt and plenty of butter or other healthy fats and serve with optional ingredients.

Chia Choco Nutty Blues Protein Pancake

3 eggs
1/4 cup Organic Blueberries (Whole Foods)
1 scoop Chocolate Protein Powder (Sun Warrior is the BOMB DOT COM)
1 tablespoon Flax Meal (Henry's)
1 tablespoon Chia Seeds (Whole Foods)
1 teaspoon of Organic Nut butter of choice (preferably roasted)

Mix all ingredients except blueberries and peanut butter. Fold in blueberries, fry it up like a pancake. Add nut butter as syrup. Nom nom nom away!

Gut healing Fiber-y Porridge

- 1/2 cup almond milk or Coconut milk or full fat organic milk
- 2 eggs
- 2 tbsp flaxseed
- 1/2 banana or 1/2 cup of berries
- 1 tbsp of grass-fed gelatin (optional)
- 1 tsp of cinnamon
- Bring milk to boil. Turn heat to medium and add eggs stirring frequently. Once it thickens, add flaxseed, banana, vanilla and cinnamon until it's like a porridge. (About 10 minutes)
- Top with almond butter, berries of choice or SMALL dash of raw honey

Coconut Macaroon Gut Healthy Porridge

- 1 cup almond milk or Coconut milk or full fat organic milk (preferably raw)
- 4 eggs
- 2 tbsp flaxseed
- 1 tablespoon of butter
- 1/2 cup unsweetened shredded coconut
- 2 tbsp of grass-fed gelatin (optional)
- 1 tsp of cinnamon
- 1 tsp of vanilla
- 2 tbsp Xyla or sweetener of choice
- Bring milk to boil. Turn heat to medium and add eggs stirring frequently.
- Pour gelatin on two tablespoons of lukewarm water in a separate bowl and let sit for a few minutes to bloom
- Once it thickens (after about 6 minutes) add flaxseed, shredded coconut, xyla, gelatin, butter, vanilla and cinnamon until it's like a porridge. (About 10 minutes)
- Top with almond butter, berries of choice or SMALL dash of raw honey

Primal Egg Muffins (good to make ahead of time and reheat)

- 1 lb ground breakfast sausage (pasture-raised, organic if possible)
- 1 dozen eggs
- Grass-fed butter, coconut oil or other fat of choice
- Salt and pepper to taste

1. Preheat oven to 350 degrees
2. Crumble and brown the pork sausage in a frying pan
or cast iron skillet.
3. In a medium/large bowl scramble one dozen large
eggs and season with salt and pepper.
4. Grease the cups of one muffin tin with oil or melted butter
5. Place equal amounts of browned sausage in the
bottoms of the muffin tins.
6. Pour the scrambled eggs evenly on top of the sausage.
The mixture will come almost to the top of the tin.
7. Cook for 20 minutes. Remove from the oven and
allow to cool for about 5 minutes.
8. Use a knife to loosen the egg muffin from the sides of
the pan.
(Good in the fridge for one week or frozen for 3 weeks)

Protein Pancakes (I like to make these ahead of time and store in the fridge.)

- 1 serving of protein powder
- 1/2 banana mashed
- 1 organic tbsp heavy whipping cream
- 2 eggs
- 1 tsp cinnamon
- Mash banana with cream, add other ingredients and cook like a pancake! Or you can bake like a muffin at 350 for about 20 minutes
- 1 tablespoon of no sugar added pure maple syrup and fruit can be added
- Optional add-ins
    - 1/4 cup of berries to batter
    - 1 tbsp apple sauce
    - 1 tbsp of almond butter and organic jam
    - 1/4 cup sliced strawberries on top
    - 1 tbsp of pumpkin puree to the batter
    - 2 tbsp of almond butter to the batter or on top
    - 1 tsp organic strawberry jam (no sugar added)
    - 1 tbsp of raisins
    - As much cinnamon as you like!

Lunch / Dinners / Sides

Perfect Salad

- 2 cups of veggies
- Unlimited mixed greens or green lettuce of choice
- 4-6 oz preferably organic free-range chicken, wild caught fish (not farm raised), organic grass-fed or pasture raised beef
- Salad dressing balsamic vinegar and olive oil

Meat Salad

- 1 cup Lettuce of choice
- Lots of olive oil + balsamic vinegar
- 6 ounces of chicken or fish or tuna or beef cooked in
- Grass-fed butter, ghee, avocado oil or coconut oil or grilled as you wish

Wedge Salad

- 1 wedge
- 1/4 cup Blue cheese
- 3 strips of bacon chopped
- 4 ounces of meat or fish of choice

Burger

- 1/4 pound organic grass-fed beef, or just organic or as natural as possible
- Lettuce cups or wedge salad
- Bacon
- Full fat organic cheese of choice
- Any vegetable fix ins you like (tomatoes, onions, pickles, mustard, organic ketchup (no sugar added)

Chicken Salad

- 4 oz chicken, cooked
- 1 tbsp full fat Greek or European yogurt
- 1 lemon, juiced
- 2 tbsp celery, chopped
- 2 tbsp carrots, shredded
- 2 tbsp onions, diced
- 1 tbsp almonds, slivered
- Pepper and sea salt to taste
- Mix everything together in a bowl. Allow to chill in fridge for an hour then serve with any lettuce you like

Peach Pecan Salad

- 1 peach, sliced
- 1 cup fresh spinach or lettuce of choice
- 1/4 cup pecans
- 4-6 oz of grilled chicken
- Dressing of choice (no sugar added no artificial flavors or additives) – I like balsamic and olive oil

Turkey breast or sliced organic turkey/chicken

- 4-6 oz of organic turkey/chicken slices
- Lettuce of choice
- Full fat cheese
- 1/4 of an avocado
- Pepperoni (organic)

Spaghetti!

- Make spaghetti sauce and meatballs of choice
- 1 spaghetti squash (2 1/2 cups)
- Cut spaghetti squash down the middle lengthwise. Place on baking sheet at cook at 350 F for 30-45 minutes. Scrape out insides with fork and place in a large mixing bowl. They will come out in long noodle like strands. Serve spaghetti sauce on top!

Chili (double recipe to serve two)

- 6 oz organic grass-fed ground beef
- 1/4 cup onion, diced
- 1/2 cup tomato, diced
- 1/2 cup kidney or black beans
- 1/2 cup bell pepper, diced
- 1 tsp. jalapeno, diced (optional)
- 1 tsp. chili powder
- 1 tsp. black pepper
- 1/2 tsp. cayenne pepper
- 1/2 cup vegetable broth
- In a medium saucepan heat beans & vegetable broth on low until they come to a simmer. Add in tomatoes and spices; stir to mix thoroughly. Meanwhile, in a medium skillet sprayed with cooking spray, cook beef on medium heat until lightly browned. Mix in onions and peppers and cook for another minute. Add contents from skillet into saucepan. Slowly add a little bit of warm water if desired to reach preferred consistency. Return to simmer. Remove from heat and serve in a bowl. Top with full fat sour cream or Greek yogurt.

Crockpot Buffalo Chicken

(I make this at least once a week and always have chicken on hand for salads, burrito bowls you name it!)

- 2-3 organic pasture raised chicken breasts
- 2 tbp Kerrygold butter or ghee, or pasture raised butter of choice
- 1/2ish cup or organic chicken stock (just fill past the breasts in the crock pot)
- 2 tablespoons of hot sauce of choice (or to taste) I loovvee O'brother chipotle hot sauce
- Salt pepper to taste
- Cook in crockpot for 6-8 hours. Shred the chicken with a fork add another tablespoon of butter, simmer another 10 mins and enjoy!!! Add some avocado, sour cream, shredded lettuce and nummmm to the errrrs.

Paleo Coconut Chicken (family fave!)

- 1 package or about 1 pound of Trader Joe's Organic Boneless Skinless Free Range Chicken Tenders (or you can cut up chicken breasts yourself)
- 1/2 cup of almond or coconut flour (I prefer almond) 2 eggs
- 1 tablespoon of organic pasture raised heavy whipping cream (optional)
- 1 Cup unsweetened shredded coconut
- Seasonings - sea salt, pepper, cayenne, paprika and lemon pepper if you so choose (play around with seasonings)
- Preheat oven to 400 degrees
- Rinse chicken
- Grease a cookie sheet with coconut oil
- Set aside three bowls - one for the flour, one for the coconut and one for the 2 eggs beat together
- Dip chicken strip in the flour, then the egg mixture then the coconut and lay strip on cookie sheet (repeat until all are coated)
- Bake at 400 for about 12-15 minutes depending on your oven. I like mine a little more well done. Mix a little ketchup with cayenne pepper and dip away!

Kale and Butternutty Delights

- 2 cups of kale (I like to buy the package at Whole Foods or Trader Joe's already cut)
- 1 cup of butternut squash cut (I like to buy the package at Whole Foods or Trader Joe's already cut)
- 1/4 cup pistachios
- Line bottom of large pan with two tablespoons of coconut oil - melt in the oven. Add the kale and butternut squash, pistachios, add another tablespoon of coconut oil and let it melt in the oven for 5 minutes. Pull it out add salt, pepper, any other seasonings you like and bake for 45 minutes at 350.

Brussels Roasted

- 1 lb of brussels washed
- 3 tablespoons of avocado or coconut oil
- Any leftover bacon grease
- Salt and pepper to taste
- 2 shakes of cayenne pepper
- 1 tbp balsamic vinegar
- 1/4 cup of crumbled goat cheese or full fat feta (optional)
- 2 tbsp lemon juice
- Mix and add to a greased baking dish, and bake for a good 30-45 minutes. Stirring every 10 or 15 minutes to brown each side. (Warning grease your baking dish well with ghee or grass-fed butter or coconut oil or it will burn and ruin the pan!)

Crockpot Taco Salad

- 1 lb grass-fed ground beef
- 1 tsp of each: chili powder, garlic powder, cumin, salt, pepper, cayenne
- Cook everything on low or medium setting stirring a few times to ensure beef is browned well
- Lettuce options:
    - 1/2 head of purple cabbage chopped + 1/2 head of green cabbage chopped
    - Cruciferous crunchy mix from Trader Joe's is also a personal fave
    - Romaine lettuce shredded
    - Add a 1/2 cup of full fat yogurt
    - Add hot sauce or fresh salsa
    - Add avocado or guacamole
    - Add the beef and serve!

Tip! If you want to save some of the beef, build the salad and add the beef on top last!

Chicken No Tortilla Soup (serves four)

- 3 large chicken breasts
- 4-6 cups of chicken stock
- 1 small onion thinly sliced
- 4-6 gloves of minced garlic
- 2 carrots diced
- 1 large Anaheim, Pasilla or Poblano pepper seeded and diced
- 2 jalapeños, seeded and diced
- 1 large can of fire roasted tomatoes
- 2 teaspoons of cumin
- 2 teaspoons of chili powder
- 2 tbsp chopped cilantro if you like
- salt and pepper to taste
- Avocado slices on top if you like or full fat sour cream
- Throw it all in the crockpot, chicken should be covered with stock. Cook on high for four hours or simmer low for eight. Shred chicken with a fork and serve!

Snack Ideas

Celery + Almond butter + Raisins

- 2 tablespoons of almond butter
- As much celery as you like
- Raisins to top

Apple sliced + 2 tbsp of almond butter

Half grapefruit + one packet of stevia + 1/4 cups of nuts

Nuts - 1/4 cup any kind but peanut + piece of fruit like a banana or peach or plum

Coffee + 2 tbsp organic heavy whipping cream + cinnamon + sea salt to taste

2 ounces of full fat organic cheese + piece of fruit

1 banana + 2 tbsp of almond butter (great dessert)

1 cup of full fat Greek or European yogurt + 1/4 cup of berries + 1/4 cup of nuts + 1/2 tsp of honey

Organic beef jerky (no sugar added)

Organic full fat cheese + piece of fruit

Turkey breast or sliced organic turkey

- Lettuce of choice
- Full fat cheese
- 1/4 of an avocado
- Pepperoni (organic)

Coconut Macaroons

- 2 cups unsweetened shredded coconut
- 1/4 teaspoon of sea salt
- 4 egg whites
- 2 tablespoons xyla sweetener (or stevia)
- 1 teaspoon vanilla
- 1 tablespoon of gelatin (optional)

1. Preheat oven to 350 degrees.
2. In a large bowl (preferably a metal bowl) beat the egg whites and salt until stiff peaks form, about 5 minutes or until they have stiff peaks.
3. Bloom your gelatin in two tablespoons of room temperature filtered water for one minute
4. Fold in the remaining ingredients until incorporated (the egg whites will deflate quite a bit).
5. Place 2 tablespoons of the batter on a parchment or silpat lined baking sheet (you can also place cookie cutters on the baking sheet and place the batter inside patting it down with a spoon to even it out. Remove the cookie cutter before baking).
6. Bake for 15 minutes or until golden.
*If you want to make 1/2 the batter chocolate macaroons, add 1 tbsp cocoa powder. If you want to make all of the macaroons chocolate, use 2 tablespoons.

Blueberry Protein Muffins

- (makes 10 muffins)
- 2 1/2 cups of protein powder
- 4 eggs
- 3 tbsp crushed walnuts
- 2 tbsp ground flaxseed
- 3/4 cup whole milk or almond milk
- 1/2 cup blueberries
- 2 tbsp of water
- 1 mashed banana
- 1/2 cup applesauce (no sugar added organic)
- 2 tbsp coconut oil
- 1 1/2 tbsp cinnamon
- 3 tsp baking powder
- Pinch of sea salt
- Combine all liquid ingredients in large bowl and mix well. Combine dry ingredients in separate bowl. Slowly add dry mixture to liquid stirring constantly. Add more milk if needed to make smooth and thick. Carefully fold blueberries into mixture. Spray cupcake wrappers lightly with cooking spray and place in muffin pan (fill the whole tin up they don't rise). Bake at 350 for 40 minutes.

Cinnamon Apple Chia Porridge (makes 4 servings)

- 1/2 cup white or black chia seeds
- 1 cup unsweetened coconut water
- 1 cup full fat unsweetened coconut milk
- 1/2 cup diced apples
- 1/2 cup raisins (optional)
- 1 tsp. cinnamon
- 1/2 tsp. nutmeg
- 1/2 tsp. sea salt
- 2 tbsp cup of pure maple syrup (no sugar or anything
- added)
- Pour chia seeds in a large mixing bowl. Add liquids and stir until well incorporated. Continue to stir for about 5 minutes off and on to make sure no clumps form. Set aside for 10-15 minutes to let the chia absorb the liquid. You will know it is ready when the consistency is of porridge. Next add remaining ingredients to the chia mixture and stir until powders and sweeteners are well incorporated. Serve immediately or store for up to 3 days.

Carrot Salad

- 1 cup carrots, grated
- 1/4 cup raisins
- 1 tbsp pecans, chopped
- 1/2 tbsp honey
- 1/2 cup of full fat Greek or European yogurt
- 1/2 lemon, juiced
- Thoroughly mix dry ingredients and honey until evenly covered. Add yogurt and squeeze lemon into mixture. Stir until completely mixed. Serve chilled.

Protein shakes

Easy. Coconut. Chocolate. Beezy. Post workout delight.
- 8 ounces of unsweetened, plain nothing added coconut water
- 2 scoops of Tera's Whey Organic Dark Chocolate Protein Powder
- Blend with 5 ice cubes and ENJOYYYY!!!

Nuts over Chocolate
- 2 cups unsweetened almond milk or 1/2 cup full fat coconut milk + 1 1/2 cup water
- 1 serving of protein powder of choice (I prefer Tera's Whey or Grass-Fed Whey)
- 2 tbsp almond butter or peanut butter (no added anything, just plain and organic)
- 1 tbsp cocoa powder
- 1/2 cup of ice

Cinnamon Lovers
- 2 cups unsweetened almond milk or 1/2 cup full fat coconut milk + 1 1/2 cup water
- 1 serving of protein powder of choice (I prefer Tera's Whey or Grass-Fed Whey)
- 1/2 tbsp ground flaxseed
- 1 - 2 tsp cinnamon depending on preferences
- Ice

Proteinaccinno (my personal fave)
- 1 cup unsweetened almond milk or 1/2 cup full fat coconut milk
- 1 cup brewed coffee chilled or room temp or two shots espresso + 1 cup water
- 1 serving of protein powder of choice (I prefer Tera's Whey or Grass-Fed Whey)
- 1 - 2 tbsp cocoa powder
- 1 tbsp coconut flakes unsweetened (optional)
- 1/2 cup of ice

Pumpkin Pie Protein Mocha
- 1/2 cup canned pumpkin
- 1 shot of espresso (or 8 ounces of coffee)
- 1/2 cup canned full fat coconut milk OR 3/4 cup of almond milk or water (add more liquid if you did the espresso)
- 1 scoop of vanilla protein powder (I used Grass-Fed Whey)
- 1 cup crushed ice
- 1 tsp ground cinnamon
- 1/2 tsp pumpkin pie spice or all spice
- 1 tbsp of cacao powder (optional, I just think everything is better with a chocolate flavor)
- 1 dash of Pasture Raised Heavy Whipping Cream

Berry Delightful

- 1/4 cup of blueberries
- 2 cups unsweetened almond milk or 1/2 cup full fat coconut milk + 1 1/2 cup water
- 1 serving of protein powder of choice (I prefer Tera's Whey or Grass-Fed Whey)
- Handful of spinach
- Ice

Popeye'd Monster

- 1/4 cup coconut water (unsweetened, plain)
- 1/2 cup water
- 1/2 frozen banana
- 1/2 cup spinach
- 1/4 avocado
- 1 tsp of stevia (optional)
- 1/4 cup hemp seeds or 1/2 tbsp of flaxseed meal (optional)

Morning Pick-me-up

- 1/2 banana
- 1/4 cup strawberries
- 1/4 cup blueberries
- 2 cups unsweetened almond milk or 1/2 cup full fat coconut milk + 1 1/2 cup water
- 1 tsp of coconut oil
- 1 serving of protein powder of choice (I prefer Tera's Whey or Grass-Fed Whey)

Skinny Green Tea Delight

- 1 cup almond milk
- 1 cup green tea (chilled or room temp)
- 1 tsp fresh ground ginger
- 1 tsp of coconut oil
- 1 serving of protein powder of choice (I prefer Tera's Whey or Grass-Fed Whey)
- 1/2 cup ice
- 1/2 tsp of stevia powder

Chocolate Covered Raspberry Mocha

- 1 1/2 cups unsweetened almond milk or 1/2 cup full fat coconut milk + 1 1/2 cup water
- 1/2 cup coffee, cold or room temp
- 1/4 cup of raspberries
- 1 tbsp cacao or unsweetened cocoa powder
- 1 serving of protein powder of choice (I prefer Tera's Whey or Grass-Fed Whey)
- 1/2 cup ice

Cookies and Coconutty Cream

- 1/2 cup full fat coconut milk + 1 1/2 cup water
- 1 serving of protein powder of choice (I prefer Tera's Whey or Grass-Fed Whey)
- 1 tbsp cacao or unsweetened cocoa powder
- 1 tbsp unsweetened carob chips or very dark chocolate chips
- 1/2 cup ice

Almond Butter Berry Time

- 2 cups unsweetened almond milk or 1/2 cup full fat coconut milk + 1 1/2 cup water
- 1 tbsp almond butter
- 1/2 cup strawberries
- Handful of spinach
- Ice

Peachy Keen

- 2 cups unsweetened almond milk or 1/2 cup full fat coconut milk + 1 1/2 cup water
- 1 peach diced
- Ice

Chocolate Almond Pie

- 2 cups unsweetened almond milk or 1/2 cup full fat coconut milk + 1 1/2 cup water
- 2 tbsp almond butter
- 1/2 frozen banana
- 1.5 tbsp cacao powder or unsweetened cocoa powder
- 1 cup water or almond milk unsweetened
- 1 serving of protein powder of choice (I prefer Tera's Whey or Grass-Fed Whey)
- 1/4 tsp. of cinnamon or to taste
- Dash of sea salt
- 1/2 tsp of stevia powder

Healthy Treats

Thin Mint Paleo Fudge (aka my favorite treat of all time)

- 2 scoops of chocolate protein powder (I used grass fed whey)
- 1 scoop of almond flour (used the same scoop from the protein powder)
- 1/3 cup of coconut oil
- 1/2 cup of nut butter of choice (I used almond butter)
- 1/4 cup of coconut flakes (unsweetened)
- 1 tb unsweetened cocoa powder
- 1 teaspoon of vanilla extract
- 1 teaspoon of peppermint extract
- Mix these ingredients
- Your consistency should be fairly moist and whipped up pretty well combined. Now pack this in a greased (optional I just think it comes out cleaner) storage system and put her in the freezer while you make the topping!

Topping
- Half of a dark chocolate bar (I used 70% Green and Black's)
- 1 tablespoon of nut butter
- Break the chocolate into pieces, add the nut butter in a microwavable bowl and melt it for like 40 seconds.
- Place it all back in the fridge and let it set for at least 30 minutes. I let mine sit overnight because it was night time anyhow and it was DELIGHTFUL in the morning!

The stupidest easiest Protein Balls of all time

- 1/2 cups of protein powder
- 1/2 cup of coconut flour
- 2 tablespoons of unsweetened cocoa powder
- 1/4 cup of hemp seeds or chia seeds
- 1/2 teaspoon of cayenne pepper
- Stir all these dry ingredients
- 2 tablespoons of coconut oil
- 1/2 tablespoon of honey
- 1/3 of cup of water incorporated very slowly, you may need more or less water, just add little by little until you have a dough you can roll into balls!

Chocolate Chip Cookies (Grain FREE)

- 1/3 cup of coconut flour
- 1/4 cup of melted coconut oil
- 1/4 cup of melted maple syrup or sweetener of choice
- 1 teaspoon of vanilla extract
- 1/4 teaspoon of sea salt
- 2 whole eggs at room temperature
- 1/3 cup of enjoy life chocolate chips, or chopped dark chocolate
- 2 tablespoons of gelatin bloomed in room temperature water
- Combine all ingredients in a mixing bowl, once a thick batter is achieved fold in chocolate chips
- Spoon out about a tablespoon and flatten into cookie shape, as they will not spread
- Bake for 12-15 minutes at 350

Beezy Protein Balls

- 1/2 cup of nut butter of choice
- 4 tbsp cocoa or cacoa powder unsweetened
- 2 tbsp of coconut oil
- 1 tbsp ground flaxseed
- 2 tbsp of unsweetened shredded coconut
- 2 tbsp of chia seeds (optional for crunchity crunch crunch and extra fiber)
- 1 scoop of chocolate protein powder
- 1 tbsp of honey or Xyla
- Sprinkle of sea salt
- Combine all in a food processor and add a tablespoon of water at a time if you need it to be more moist. Roll into 1-inch or so balls, I made 16 balls.

Chocolate Gooey Nut Butter Mug cake

- 2 tablespoons almond flour
- 1 tablespoon flax meal
- 1/2 tablespoon of gelatin or 1 scoop of protein powder
- 1/4 teaspoon baking soda
- 3 tablespoons of milk of choice
- 1/2 teaspoon of honey or stevia to taste
- Spray your favorite mug with cooking spray (preferably coconut oil spray) mix all dry ingredients, add the wet and mix well
- Add one tablespoon of nut butter RIGHT in the middle of your batter without mixing
- Cook for 30-60 seconds depending on your microwave
- Grab a spoon and devour

Cinnamon Protein Bread

- 2 Cups Almond Flour
- 2 tbsp of gelatin or replace 1/4 cup of flour with protein powder of choice
- 1/8 Tsp Sea Salt
- 1/2 Tbsp Baking Soda
- 1 Tbsp Baking Powder
- 2 Tbsp Unsweetened Applesauce
- 1 Tbsp Unsweetened Coconut Milk or plain all raw milk
- 1 Tbsp Honey
- 2 Tbsp Cinnamon
- 2 Eggs
- 4 tbsp Ground Flax Seed
- Topping - 1 tablespoon of honey melted in full fat organic yogurt

Apple Cinnamon Nutty Muffins

- 5 eggs
- 1 cup homemade or organic no sugar added store bough applesauce
- 1 cups of nut butter of choice
- ½ cup coconut flour
- 2-3 TBSP cinnamon
- 1 tsp baking soda
- 1 tsp vanilla
- ¼ cup coconut oil
- 2 Tbsp honey (optional) or coconut sugar or Xyla
- 1 tbsp of gelatin bloomed in 2 tablespoons of room temp water (optional)

1. Preheat the oven to 400 degrees F
2. Grease a muffin pan with coconut oil or butter (grease them well!)
3. Put all ingredients into a medium sized bowl, mix very well. I like to use my counter top kitchen aid mixer, but you could use an immersion blender too. Just want it really mixed really well.
4. Let it sit 5 minutes.
5. Use ⅓ cup measure to spoon into muffin tins.
6.. Bake 12-15 minutes until starting to brown and not soft when lightly touched on the top.
7. Let cool and drizzle with honey and serve!

Brownie My Heart

- 2 Small Ripe Bananas (blended in a food processor to make creamy)
- 3 Tbsp Ground Flax Seed
- 3 Tbsp Chia Seeds
- 2 Packets Truvia or Stevia
- 1/2 Tsp Baking Powder
- 1/2 Tsp Baking Soda
- 2 Scoops chocolate whey protein powder
- 1 tablespoon Unsweetened Cocoa Powder
- 1 teaspoon Vanilla Extract
- Mix dry ingredients. Mix wet ingredients. Fold together everything and bake at 350 for 10-12 minutes.

Beezy Sauce! Aka Chocolate Heaven

- 2 cups unsweetened coconut flakes
- 2 tablespoons cocoa powder
- 1 tablespoon honey or blend in 4 dates or low carb go for 2 tablespoons of Xyla
- 1 teaspoon sea salt (or to taste)

Place nuts in a food processor or Vitamix. Process for 7-10 minutes, scraping down the sides as necessary. The nuts will first get powdery, then pasty, and then start to form a butter. Process until the nuts have turned smooth and dripping. Remove from the Vitamix or food processor and stir in the remaining ingredients. Store in an airtight jar.

Blonde Beezy Bars!

Dry Ingredients

- 6 scoops of Chocolate Protein Powder (I used It's About Time Whey Chocolate Peanut Butter
- 1/4 cup cacao powder
- 3 tbsp flax meal
- 3 tbsp shredded coconut
- 2 tbsp coconut sugar or xyla (could use teaspoon of stevia)
- 1/4 tsp baking soda
- 1 tablespoon of grass-fed gelatin (optional)
- Pinch of salt

Wet Ingredients

- 4 eggs
- 1 cup high quality almond milk
- 1 cup full fat organic greek yogurt (I always prefer full fat yogurt because it tends to have less sugar and less processed or unsweetened organic apple sauce)
- 1/4 cup of berries
- 5 drops liquid stevia
- 1 teaspoon vanilla extract
- 1 teaspoon almond extract
- Mix the dry ingredients in one bowl, and the wet in another bowl, then mix all together and bake in a greased pyrex dish or baking pan at 350 for about 8-12 minutes depending on your oven! Just keep checking those nuggets.

Frosting (blend everything in a blender)

- 8 oz Greek yogurt
- 1/2 cup of coconut milk (organic straight from the can)
- 1/2 banana
- 1 tsp vanilla
- 1 tsp of cinnamon
- Add as many shakes of sprinkles as you like (the only non clean ingredient but OH so delicious)

Pour the icing all over the cake and then put it in the freezer for 30-45 minutes to set. If you are traveling somewhere to deliver the cake I'd say 45 minutes. Cut into 16 squares after you set the frosting. Store pan in the fridge!

OR

You could also just keep the icing in a bowl and add it as you eat the cake as it will get melty!

Coconut Protein Cookies

- Dry ingredients
- 3/4 cup of almond flour
- 1/4 cup of flax meal
- 4 scoops of vanilla whey protein
- 1/2 cup unsweetened shredded coconut
- 1/4 cup of Xyla (you could use stevia too)
- 1/2 teaspoon of baking soda
- 1/4 teaspoon of salt
-

Wet Ingredients (mash this up in a separate bowl)

- 4 egg whites or 3 whole eggs
- 1 teaspoon of almond extract
- 1 teaspoon of vanilla extract
- 1/2 cup of almond butter (or your favorite nut butter)
- Combine everything together and bake at 350 for about 12 minutes.

Low Carb Chocolate Chip Cookies!

- 3 eggs
- 1⁄2 cup softened butter
- 1 teaspoon vanilla extract
- 1⁄2 teaspoon cinnamon
- 1⁄2 teaspoon nutmeg
- 3⁄4 cup birch xylitol or 2 teaspoon stevia powder extract
- (Or 3/4 cup coconut sugar for Paleo)
- 1⁄3 cup coconut flour
- 1⁄2 teaspoon baking soda
- 1⁄2 teaspoon sea salt
- 1 cup almond meal
- 4 ounces unsweetened dark chocolate, chopped
- Preheat the oven to 350° F.
- Mix the eggs, palm shortening or butter, vanilla, cinnamon, nutmeg, and sweetener in a large bowl.
- Sift the coconut flour into a small bowl then add the baking soda, salt, and almond flour.
- Combine the two mixtures and add the chocolate chunks.
- Place parchment paper on cookie sheets.
- Spoon the dough on the cookie sheet in 1-inch mounds.
- Bake for 15-17 minutes until browned.

Chocolate Coconut Brownies

- 8 egg yolks
- 1 avocado
- 2 tablespoons of gelatin
- 2 cups shredded coconut
- 2 tablespoons coconut oil
- 1/4 teaspoon sea salt
- 2 tablespoons xyla
- 1 teaspoon vanilla
- 2 tablespoons cocoa powder

Paleo Blueberry Lemon Muffins

Wet Stuff
- 3 eggs
- 2 tablespoons of coconut oil
- 2 tablespoons of grass fed butter
- 2 tablespoons of coconut butter (could just use another tablespoon of butter instead)
- 1/4 cup of honey or unsweetened grade a maple syrup
- 1 teaspoon of vanilla extract
- 1 lemon (juice + zest)
- Combine all your wet stuff in a bowl (may need to melt your oils and butters)

Dry Stuff
- 1 cup of almond flour
- 1 teaspoon of sea salt
- 1/4 cup of coconut flakes (could use more or omit)
- 1/4 tsp of baking soda

Mix all your dry stuff, then combine with wet stuff and make a batter then fold in 2 cups of frozen or fresh blueberries. (If frozen allow to thaw for 30 minutes at room temperature.) You can make 6 giant muffins, or spoon 12 small muffins filling your muffin tins about half the way. Bake at 350 for 20-30 minutes if you make 6 big boys.

Skinny Mini Cinnamony Yogurt

- 1/2 cup of full fat organic yogurt
- 1-2 teaspoons of cinnamon (I like mine real cinnamony like)
- Shake of sea salt (optional)
- Blend and enjoy

Cookies. Mother effing. Cookies.

- 4 scoops tera's whey dark chocolate
- 1 cup almond flour
- 2 cups unsweetened shredded coconut
- 1/4 cup cacao powder or unsweetened cocoa powder
- 1/4 cup flax meal
- 1/4 cup coconut sugar or xyla
- 1/4 teaspoon sea salt
- mix all these dry goods
- add 4 eggs
- 2 tablespoons of coconut oil
- 1 teaspoon of vanilla
- Bake at 350 for 8-11 minutes (I say undercook em for a good chewy bite!)

Sweet Potato Cookies

- 2 tbsp coconut oil
- 2 eggs
- 1 teaspoon cinnamon
- 1.5 cups almond flour
- 1 baked and soft sweet potato
- 1 tbsp raw maple syrup
- 2 tbsp flax meal
- 1/4 tsp baking powder
- 2 tbsp almond butter
- Grease cookie sheet with coconut oil
- Mix and bake at 350 for about 25 minutes.
- You can flip over halfway through for the best consistency.
- Makes about a dozen.

Low Carb Chocolate Coconut Ice Cream

- 1/2 cup of full fat coconut milk from the can (skip the carton stuff too many fillers and crap you don't need)
- 1 tbsp of unsweetened cocoa or cacao powder
- 1 tbsp of organic heavy whipping cream (optional makes it whip it and creamy real nice like)
- 1 teaspoon of honey

Whip it up for 2 minutes and place it in the freezer for 20-30 minutes more if you want it frozen less if you want it like pudding

Sips'n'such

Detox Tea

- 2 bags Green Tea
- Juice of one lemon
- 2 tablespoons apple cider vinegar
- Ginger

Butter Cup of Joe

- 1 - 2 cups hot coffee or 1-2 shots espresso + 8 ounces hot water
- 1 tablespoon of high quality pasture raised butter or ghee
- 1 tablespoon of coconut oil or MCT oil
- Shakes of sea salt
- Shakes of cinnamon
- 1 teaspoon of unsweetened cocoa powder (optional)
- 1 shake of cayenne pepper

Kombucha in a wine glass

- 4 ounces of sparkling mineral water
- 4 ounces of kombucha

Ginger Spice Slice

The goal is to make this every week and chew these gut loving babies as needed, preferably before meals. Should be eaten before every meal during gut cleanse. You do not drink this solution.

- Squeeze 1/2 cup of fresh lemon juice into a cup, jar or pitcher
- Cut up a knob of fresh ginger into thin one inch strips
- Add 1/2 teaspoon of sea salt then stir

12.
RESOURCES

Here are my favorite resources, websites and tools! xo

WEBSITES

The Eating Academy - http://eatingacademy.com/

Nutrition Science Initiative - http://nusi.org/

The Weston A. Price Foundation - http://www.westonaprice.org/

Mark's Daily Apple - http://www.marksdailyapple.com/

Wellness Mama - http://wellnessmama.com/

Chris Kesser - http://chriskresser.com/

Tim Ferriss - http://fourhourworkweek.com/blog/

Paleo Chef - http://paleochef.com/

January Wellness - http://www.januarywellness.com/

PRODUCTS

Ferrofood - http://amzn.to/1vjZgGr

Gelatin - http://amzn.to/1xATAoP

Apple Cider Vinegar - http://amzn.to/1ycPBSW

Magnesisum - http://amzn.to/1th6eYw

L-Glutamine - http://amzn.to/1th6nuO

Probiotic - http://amzn.to/1uCBDnI

Digestive Enzyme - http://amzn.to/1yTc5Hb

Aloe Vera Juice - http://amzn.to/1xYdoaQ

Dry Brush - http://amzn.to/1rd79y0

Evan Healy Skincare (THE BEST!!!!) - http://amzn.to/11Vs8cf

Fermented Cod Liver Oil - http://amzn.to/1th5XEW

Dandy Blend - http://amzn.to/1th60kb

NRG Matrix - http://amzn.to/11VswaP

Nourishing Traditions Cookbook - http://amzn.to/1uUsA6G

Weleda Toothpaste - http://amzn.to/1zr1SBO

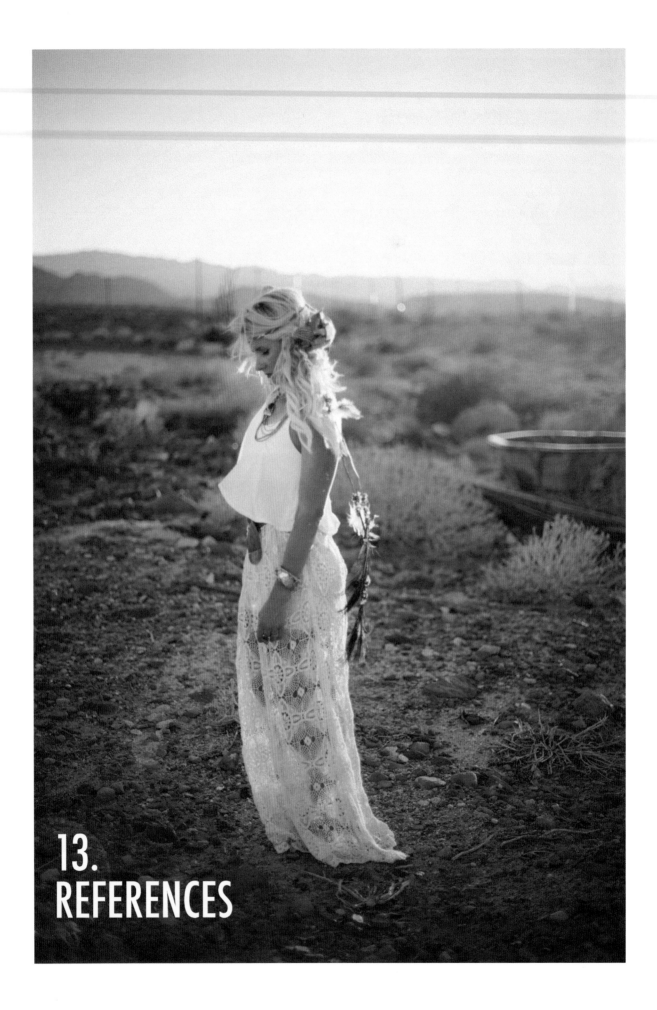

13.
REFERENCES

REFERENCES

1. Dr. Mercola - http://articles.mercola.com/sites/articles/archive/2013/06/20/gut-brain-connection.aspx

2. "Tight Junctions, Intestinal Permeability, and Autoimmunity Celiac Disease and Type 1 Diabetes Paradigms." *PMC*. June 16, 2010.

3. Fallon, Sall and Enig, Mary. www.price-pottenger.org. Price-Pottenger Foundation Website

4. The autoimmune bases of infertility and pregnancy loss. *Epub*. Jan 27, 2012.

5. Probiotic lactobacillus and estrogen effects on vaginal epithelial gene expression responses to Candida albicans. *J Biomed Sci*. June 20,2012

6. Beating the Food Giants. http://www.whale.to/v/stitt_b1.html

7. The mislabelling of deoxycorticosterone: making sense of corticosteroid structure and function. *J. Endocrinol.* October, 2011.

8. Dietary cholesterol and coronary artery disease: a systematic review. *Curr Atheroscler.* November 11, 2009.

9. Understanding Cholesterol. Harvard Health.

10. Effect of hydration status on thirst, drinking, and related hormonal responses during low-intensity exercise in the heat. *JAP.* July, 2004.

11. Effects of Dietary Composition on Energy Expenditure During Weight-Loss Maintenance. *JAMA.* June 27, 2012.

12. Eating Academy. Website. http://eatingacademy.com/glossary

13. Mark's Daily Apple. Website. http://www.marksdailyapple.com/is-wheat-addictive/#axzz3KL99C2n7

14. Effect of feeding systems on omega-3 fatty acids, conjugated linoleic acid and trans fatty acids in Australian beef cuts: potential impact on human health. *Asia Pac J Clin Nutr.* 2006

15. Protein: metabolism and effect on blood glucose levels. *Diabetics Educ.* November, 1997.

16. Low-fat dietary pattern and weight change over 7 years: the Women's Health Initiative Dietary Modification Trial. *JAMA.* January 4, 2006.

17. The Awful Truth About Eating Grains. Article. http://articles.mercola.com/sites/articles/archive/2008/01/02/truth-about-eating-grains.aspx

18. 7 Reasons to Eat More Fat. Article. http://articles.mercola.com/sites/articles/archive/2009/09/22/7-reasons-to-eat-more-saturated-fat.aspx

19. Effect of processing on contents and relationships of mineral elements of milk. Department of Food Hygiene and Technology, University of Córdoba, Medina Azahara 9, 14005 Córdoba, Spain

20. HIIT vs. CARDIO. http://www.unm.edu/~lkravitz/Article%20folder/HIITvsCardio.html

Printed in Great Britain
by Amazon.co.uk, Ltd.,
Marston Gate.